CLEA

THE HOLISTIC DI
for mind, b

C000008564

FAITH CANTER

Wishing you HEALTH & HAPPINESS

Faith x

EMPOWERED
BOOKS

Published in 2016 by Empowered Books

ISBN Paperback: 978-0-9957047-0-1
Ebook: 978-0-9957047-1-8

A CIP catalogue copy of this book can be found in the British Library.

Published with the help of Indie Authors World

IndieAuthors
World

DEDICATION

To me dear friend Lucy.

You are without a doubt one of the most authentic, honest and caring people I have had the pleasure to not only meet but call my friend. Thank you for always shining so brightly and encouraging me to do the same.

To all of you amazing people out there who have had the courage to say 'Enough is enough, and things are going to change!' You guys rock and inspire me every day!

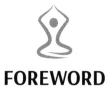

FOREWORD

Every now and again a book comes along that changes your life – this is one of those books.

How do I know?

Because I've been through this Cleanse Program, and it gave me my life back!

I used to think that I looked after myself well – eating and drinking sensibly, exercising regularly, meditating and using various other practices to put myself in the best place to enjoy life physically, emotionally, and spiritually.

But last year my body decided otherwise. It had had enough.

I'd become physically exhausted and most days was struggling to get out of bed. Headaches and migraines made regular appearances, often accompanied with dizzy spells. My skin was blotchy. I was experiencing unusual mood swings. And my weight was going in the wrong direction – even though I was following what I thought was a healthy diet.

What was happening? It didn't make sense.

My doctor had briskly dismissed my concerns, suggesting I simply needed to get more sleep. But I knew something else was wrong, and so booked a session with Faith.

5

Gosh, I'm so glad I did!

I had no idea what to expect but was ready to listen.

I was so desperate for the energetic and optimistic version of me to return, I was ready to do whatever I needed to do for this to happen.

What did I need to do?

I left armed with lists of goodies to buy, and notes on how to change my diet and heal my body – essentially, the contents of this book.

I'd never felt so compelled to take control of my health, and I started this Cleanse Program the very next day.

Initially some of the new ingredients seemed odd, but I persevered and was pleasantly surprised at how much easier it was to stick to the program than I'd thought it would be.

You see, Faith, suggests an approach that sets you up to succeed.

Rather than immediately cutting out the 'bad' stuff, as many 'diets' do, Faith takes you through a kinder process of nurturing a positive mindset, overcoming emotional resistance, and changing eating and lifestyle habits week by week – so you're more likely to make the changes your body needs.

After only a couple of weeks following this program, I felt so much better.

Seriously, I had lots more energy and my enthusiasm for life had returned.

Phew, what a relief!

But the best bit is that now, a year later, I'm much better at taking care of myself and listening to my body – recognising when I need to rest, modifying my eating, or stepping up other health practices to restore a healthy blend of chemicals and hormones in my body.

How would you feel, if you were healthier?

It is possible for you to start healing your body today.

If you're unsure how, Faith has written this practical step-by-step guide for you.

It really is a fantastic resource for anyone who'd like more energy, to lose weight, or is looking for a holistic approach to healing a lingering health issue.

But don't just trust my word. Try it for yourself!

With love,

Alisoun x

Alisoun Mackenzie

Business Mentor, Speaker and Author of Amazon Bestseller *Heartatude, The 9 Principles of Heart-Centered Success*

TESTIMONIALS FOR CHANGE

'You did a great job, Faith. The cleanse/detox was much more fun with your support, and I feel a lot wiser because of it and was able to stick to it that bit better because of you. As a coach myself, I wasn't always sure about the area of health, and I feel I know a lot more now; so more rounded in my own knowledge, and less rounded round the middle, as I'm a few lbs lighter now.'

Lester, Edinburgh

'I can thoroughly recommend Faith's Cleanse Program. It's almost like Faith is walking personally next to you and holding your hand every step of the way. The most nurturing, holistic, and self-supportive program I have done in a very long time. I have definitely seen the results and positive changes in my life. Thank you so very much, Faith, you really are a miracle worker.'

Tracy, Bristol

'I took part in Faith's cleanse at the beginning of this year. I very much welcomed this as a great opportunity to reset and rebalance my whole system. At the end of the cleanse, I felt better and clearer both mentally and physically. I am now continuing with choosing natural sources of sugar only, and avoiding processed and hidden sugars. Not because I *should* but because I personally experienced how great it feels. Thank you for all you do, Faith!'

Veronika, Edinburgh

'On doing the cleanse, the first benefit I had was within 2 days when I stopped getting indigestion which I had suffered from every day for over 2 years. It has not recurred. I'm so grateful to Faith for introducing me to this type of detox.'

Pam, Edinburgh

'Within days of starting Faith's 'Cleanse' program, I had MUCH more energy. That in itself was great. However, after a few weeks, I noticed a massive benefit – chronic joint pain (affecting daily activities) drastically reduced, and I could walk almost pain-free. I've found that by following Faith's recommendations I've curbed sugar cravings and no longer consume sugary/processed foods, resulting in weight loss without diet! I no longer feel bloated and I actually feel the best I've felt in years! The steps are easy to follow and any questions are swiftly answered. I'd recommend anyone contemplating a detox to try Faith's program. I'm so glad I took that initial decision to "get on board". Thanks again – this has literally changed my life.

May, Edinburgh

CONTENTS

About the Author

Having recovered from ME/CFS and a whole host of other health concerns, using a whole life approach to detoxing mind, body, home and environment, I wrote my first book, *Living a Life Less Toxic*, to assist others in regaining their own health and vitality. My own recovery and that of my clients was what inspired me to write that book. What I didn't realise, however, was that the journey to publishing it would be just as healing as the journey that had led to the book being written in the first place.

The Universe conspired – sometimes it felt like against me, but now I realise it was with me –to publish *Living a Life Less Toxic*, because from the moment I decided to write it everything fell into place and I ended up winning a self-publishing contract from Hay House Publishing UK with their sister company, Balboa Press. However, I wasn't to know that this process was also to be part of my healing journey, for in the months that followed I slowly but surely felt like I was losing the plot! Me, who had it all sorted, had healed myself, was helping others...lost the plot (all over again)!

I suddenly doubted myself again, feared putting myself 'out there' in the big scary world, and was anxious about the criticism I thought might come of me and my baby (book). Through the months of self-doubt during the publishing process, I hurt, I healed, and I learned to live more in harmony with myself and life itself. I realised that everything going on in my life was showing up as invitations to resolve things for me at an even deeper level than before. As I became more aware of this concept, I was not only able to resolve my own 'stuff' in a much quicker and kinder way, but I noticed this was also happening for my clients as well.

The more I resolved my own stuff, the more I helped others, and the more of this book (that you hold in your hands) started to take form. Some of the same things feature here as in my first book, but at a much deeper and more healing level. I hope you find this book as helpful as I did in writing it.

Life really does give us everything we need, even if it doesn't feel like it at the time!

Much love,

Faith

You can contact me by email at

faith@faithcanter.com

or at my website

www.faithcanter.com

Introduction: What is Cleanse?

You have either picked this book up to address your health or to lose weight. Well, it's really all about having harmonious health... period!

What I mean by this is that balancing your weight, your hormones, your mood, your skin, etc, etc, is a by-product of true health and harmony within your body and mind. This is the same for many health conditions and concerns, many of which you may feel are incurable or unrelated to why you want to take part in the Cleanse program. I've lost count of the number of clients who come to me for one problem and, when I have 'prescribed' this holistic detox program, they find their original concerns and many other areas they didn't come to me for have cleared up as well.

Having taken hundreds of clients through this six-week holistic detox program, I know how important it is to nourish and nurture both body and mind when detoxing from toxic thoughts, feelings, bodies, homes, and environments. Detox programs that don't nourish and nurture often leave us feeling depleted; we don't stick to them, or we end up embarking on another one a few months down the line as we are back to square one again.

You'll find this program is unlike any other detox you have come across before. It's totally and utterly nurturing in every single way.

When cleansing body and mind together, we learn new ways of thinking about ourselves, our lives, and our bodies. This creates healthy and nurturing ways to live our lives, not just for the next six weeks but into the future as well.

You don't have to spend lots of time and energy on this process. You simply start by following this six-week *Cleanse* program that will help you to achieve a more harmonious and healthy body and mind. After this stage, you can still enjoy the foods and drinks you like and do the things you want to do, but you simply continue with some of the items in this program as a sort of maintenance dose of health and harmony. This way, you won't find yourself feeling the need to do another detox, cleanse, or diet in another few months' time.

By putting a little time aside to address your overall health and wellbeing in a holistic and harmonious way like this, you can look after yourself and your family more easily. You may become more productive at work, you will no longer wake up exhausted, your weight will balance out to a healthy level, and you may be able to eliminate many pills and potions you have been taking/using. Being healthy isn't just about changing your diet; it's about reducing your toxic load, both mentally and physically.

Over the next six weeks I'll be guiding you along your very own do-it-yourself holistic detox program and on to better health, harmony, and wellbeing. What have you got to lose? Health and harmony could literally be just around the corner...now that's pretty awesome, wouldn't you say?

How to Use this Book

Use this book in the order it is set out. Bish, bash, bosh!

Okay, so there may be a little bit more to it than that...but you'll be pleased to know, not much!

Start with the preparation station section, as this will set you up for what's to come. It'll make sure you're fully prepared for the Cleanse program. It explains how to get focused, what to purchase, what to use up or give away, and how to get into a nourishing and healing headspace. This is the fundamental foundation for the program, and will help you understand what's going on and why throughout the rest of the book. Of course, it will also help you maintain this harmonious way of life.

Section two is the six-week Cleanse program itself. Again, this is best to do in the order it is presented, to minimise detox symptoms and to support your mind and body through these nourishing changes. Of course, if you feel you are already have a fairly nourishing and healthy life, you could skip to week three and work from there, but, where possible, it's best to do the whole program as it's laid out within the pages of this book.

Section three is continuing this healthy and harmonious way of life after the program. You'll see you can go on to enjoy your life yet still maintain great health and wellbeing, without having to repeatedly do detoxes, diets, or cleanses. As long as you support the body and mind in a nourishing and harmonious way to minimise the impact of toxins you may take on board, both mentally and physically, you can have a full, fun, and healthy life.

Last, but not least, section four is packed full of recipes for making your own nourishing meals (both cooked and raw), smoothies, teas, and probiotic fermented foods and drinks. Please feel free to dip in and out of this delicious section as and when you feel the call to create something nourishing, cleansing, and yummy to consume.

Section One:
The Preparation Station

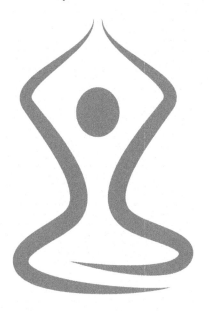

Chapter 1: Get Focused

Why haven't other programs, diets, or detoxes worked for you, and why have you picked up a book about another one? There are several reasons. Firstly, it's unlikely you were focusing on health; more so, you may have been focusing on weight loss or just wanting to feel a little less toxic after a bit of a blowout. Secondly, most detoxes focus on short term goals, they're quick fixes and are not about long term lifestyle changes for long and lasting results. Finally, and most importantly, it's unlikely those other detoxes helped you get into the right frame of mind to stick to the program. Not only this, but they probably also failed to help you continue nourishing yourself way beyond the program, otherwise you wouldn't be reading about this program. And lastly, the other programs may not have covered the fact that there are many mind-based causes to many physical issues you may be struggling with which need to be resolved for health, happiness, and harmony within body and mind.

It doesn't have to be a battle of wills, you don't need to fight against yourself, and you really can achieve everything you set out to achieve during the next six weeks! Getting focused for what's to come is quite simple. First, we start by seeing what may be causing conflict for you when you embark on this or any period of change.

By this, I mean that you probably want to improve your health or lose weight, but...

1. You hate healthy food.

2. You haven't got time to be healthy.

3. You can't live without chocolate.

4. You enjoy a few boozy drinks.

5. Diets don't work for you.

6. You and exercise do not see eye-to-eye.

7. You can't afford to change to new healthy habits.

8. You enjoy a nice takeaway a little too often.

9. You feel you already don't eat much.

10. Everyone in your family is weighty.

If your reasons for not getting healthy are like any of the above, then you're in the right place! We will create a new nourishing life together right here, in the next six weeks.

First things first, let's deal with that pesky mind! We both know it's the mind that's been holding you back. It's the mind that's telling you that you don't have time, you simply must have that takeaway, or that all healthy food sucks! The mind can literally play mind games with us and we let it, not because we are weak, but because we don't understand that it's simply running programs based on our beliefs and habits, whether they're true or not.

What I'd like you to do now is write down all your beliefs around getting fit and healthy. Be REALLY truthful (it's the only way to resolve them). Even if the truth seems silly or even not relevant, write it all down, get it all out. There's no prizes for being cagey, but you'll find many for being truthful. These could be any of the items in the list above, or any of the following:

1. I'll never lose weight.
2. I put the weight on during my pregnancy, and everyone knows that it's hard to lose pregnancy weight.
3. I'm not well enough to eat healthily.
4. I'm too tired to change my routine.
5. I'm too stressed to eat better.
6. My husband/wife does all the cooking and they won't eat healthy food.
7. Yoga, running, and exercise in general is sooooo boring!
8. I'll never be beautiful.
9. I don't want to be seen.
10. My weight is protecting/supporting me.
11. Even when I lose weight, it never stays off.
12. I'll never get well.
13. I'll never have the energy to do this.
14. I'll never have enough hours in the day.
15. I want this so badly, but I don't want to change my life.
16. I don't have the willpower.
17. I hate myself, so what's the point?
18. Why do I struggle so much with these things when others seem to find them so easy?
19. I'll never be satisfied with healthy food.
20. No-one understands how I feel.

Add as many things to your list as you can think of. Don't stop until you have every tiny little belief around being healthy down on your piece(s) of paper. These are what we call limiting beliefs; these are holding you back from the nourishing lifestyle you deserve. You can't simply not think of them and hope that they'll go away...they don't! They will keep niggling at you, and these are the reasons why willpower alone almost never works. They create negative pathways in the brain that you then reinforce by continually focusing on them or even playing the ignoring game. These then create chemical reactions in the body to hinder your progress, to keep you stuck, unhealthy, fat/thin, tired, and lacking in whatever you feel is missing to make you happy.

So, the first step on this nourishing journey is to resolve these limiting beliefs, and thus throw the shutters wide open to health.

I know you might not want to 'go there', dig deep, or be thrown in at the deep end, but if that's the case I'd put money on the fact that this is the stuff that's been holding you back from health during all the other detoxes, diets, or programs that you've tried before. These are the things that underlie your happiness, these are the real reasons you are content just the way you are. It's not your weight, health, job, relationship, or home, as these come and go throughout your life. It's that uneasiness, that little voice, that's where it all stems from. Pretending not to think about something does not make it go away; it causes conflict within the mind and body, and this then causes all manner of mental and physical reactions to happen within you. It's time to put on your big girl pants (or boxers) and give what I am about to tell you a real go. Let's once and for all create the health, harmony, and happiness you deserve!

Now that you have your list of limiting beliefs, let's start to resolve them. I want to make something very clear here: you don't need fixing or changing. You are (even if you don't believe this just yet) a totally perfect, beautiful human being! We are just going to work on resolving what's holding you back from realising this and obtaining your health goals.

And the first way we are going to start resolving it is by something called tapping/emotional freedom technique (EFT). This is an all-time favourite of mine, and can be used for so many different things. Anything from day-to-day stresses and anxieties, phobias, and deep-seated memories from childhood, from traumas, or from things you weren't even aware that your subconscious mind is playing in the background.

Tapping works by verbalising what you are internalising, whilst tapping on meridian (acupressure/acupuncture) points throughout the body. This releases blockages, emotions, energy, pain, heartache, stress – you name it! I'm about to explain the technique to you, but I want you to remember the following…

1. Don't get caught up in 'doing it right', just do whatever you can whenever you can. Every little tap, no matter how small, really does help!

2. If you can't manage the whole routine, can't remember it, or are too tired for it, just do what you can when you can. Every little tap, no matter how small, really does help!

3. If you are not sure what to work on or how, just tap on one of your limiting beliefs or the fact that you are not sure

what to work on, and see what happens. Every little tap, no matter how small, really does help!

4. If you get upset, anxious, or even angry whilst tapping, don't stop, keep going, work with the emotions, where you are feeling them, how, what colour are they, or any random thoughts at all that come up, just keep going. Every little tap, no matter how small, really does help!

5. If you are thinking about it in your mind, then it will be affecting your health in some way or another, so tap on it. Every little tap, no matter how small, really does help!

6. Saying all the positive affirmations or words in the world won't help if internally you are thinking the opposite, like 'I hate myself, I'm fat/thin, ugly, tired, ill, in pain'. Verbalise your internal thoughts whilst tapping, as this allows you to use these beliefs for healing, rather than repeating them over and over again for no benefit at all. Every little tap, no matter how small, really does help!

7. When you feel your thoughts (like when you feel discomfort in your chest when stressed, etc), tap on those. You don't have to label them, just be with them, tap on them and then let them go. Every little tap, no matter how small, really does help!

8. If you are not ready to deal with something, then tap on being open and ready to address it the next time around. This gives the subconscious permission to work on it in the future. Every little tap, no matter how small, really does help!

9. If you feel stressed or anxious about tapping, then tap on the stress and anxiety around tapping and not on the limiting belief itself. There's no point in forcing yourself to tap when you are resisting it; it will be counterproductive, and you will be less likely to tap next time. Resolve the conflict around why you don't want to tap first. This might be things like: you don't get it; you don't believe it will work; you feel silly; or you don't know if you are doing it right. Whatever the reason, tap on those first. Every little tap, no matter how small, really does help!

10. When you realise that you are deep in thought, tap! You will never resolve a problem in the same head space that created it, so speak your truth, tap it out, and let it go. At this stage the answer will come, or you simply won't care about whatever the question was. Either way, it won't be going around and around in your head, causing stress, anxiety and disharmony. Every little tap, no matter how small, really does help!

By now you should get the picture that any tapping helps, you can't tap too much or on the wrong things, the only thing that would be wrong would be to not tap at all! Every little tap, no matter how small, really does help!

Resolution through tapping:

1. Which of your limiting beliefs is bothering you the most? Be specific, add as much detail around this belief/event/feeling as possible. Does it feel like a colour? Can you feel it in your body somewhere? Does it make you feel sick to the stomach, tight in the chest, tearful, drained, scared, etc?

2. For the sake of this exercise, let's name your limiting belief 'I'll never be well'. Rate the intensity of your feelings about your chosen belief on a scale of 0-10 (10 being the worst).

3. Next put together a set-up phrase. The set-up phrase focuses the mind on the belief. (If you prefer, and if you find the set-up phrase confusing, you can miss this stage out until you get the hang of the rest of the sequence.)

Here are some options for the set-up phrase you can use:

Even though I feel I'll never be well, *I deeply and completely love and accept myself.*

Even though I feel I'll never be well, *I am willing to seek out harmonious ways to live.*

Even though I feel I'll never be well, *I love and accept my young self.*

Even though I feel I'll never be well, *I honour myself with this nurturing time of healing.*

Even though I feel I'll never be well, *I can choose to be kinder to myself.*

Even though I feel I'll never be well, **I** *am open to loving and accepting myself.*

Even though I feel I'll never be well, *I can accept that this is just the way I feel right now.*

Even though I feel I'll never be well, *I am open to living more from the heart than the head.*

Note: If you are struggling with believing any of the above set-up phrases then you may want to add them to your limiting beliefs list, and do some tapping on resolving the conflict you have with believing them. Either way, don't get hung up on them.

4. To perform the set-up phase, tap on the karate chop point (see diagram below) and repeat your chosen set-up phrase three times: Even though I feel I'll never be well, I...

5. Tap on the below points, roughly ten times each (starting with the top of the head and working down) while repeating reminder phrases. Reminder phrases are your limiting beliefs around whatever it is you are working on. This could be how it is affecting you, mentally, physically, and spiritually. You could say things like:

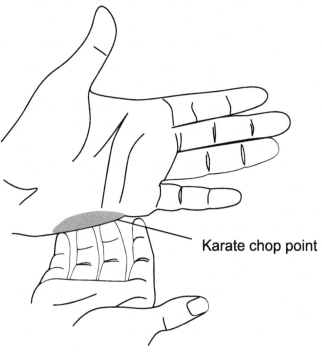

Karate chop point

I feel like I'll never get well because I've been unwell for so long.

I feel like I'll never get well because others haven't.

I feel like I'll never get well because I've tried everything.

I feel like I'll never get well because my life sucks.

I feel like I'll never get well because I don't want to go back to the life I had before.

I feel like I'll never get well because I can't deal with my life.

I feel like I'll never get well because of the people/stress/ places in my life.

This feeling feels like it will never end.

This feeling feels like a large knot in the tummy.

This feeling feels like a big black cloud hanging over me.

This feeling feels like pressure.

This feeling feels like I am being dragged under.

This feeling feels like it's stuck in my throat.

This feeling started after...

This feeling reminds me of...

This feeling feels like...

I give myself permission to heal (this one is super important).

I give myself permission to be kinder to myself.

I give myself permission to live in health and harmony once more.

6. Basically, say anything that pops into your mind. No matter how irrelevant it feels, you should tap on it. It's especially important to try and think of the first time you felt like this and work from there, as that's probably the core reason that's holding you back from healing.

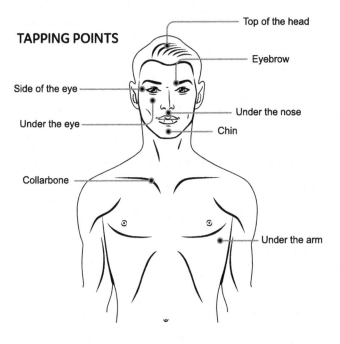

TAPPING POINTS

Top of the head

Eyebrow

Side of the eye

Under the nose

Under the eye

Chin

Collarbone

Under the arm

7. After a couple of rounds of tapping, reassess the intensity level of whatever it is you are working on. If the number has dropped, then you're on the right track. If it hasn't, then perhaps this isn't the core issue. Try focusing on the first

time you ever remember feelings similar to the ones you're focussing on, and give that a go.

8. If it has dropped, but is not down to zero, refocus on your issue and continue tapping, saying things like:

These remaining feelings around not becoming well again are...

These remaining feelings around not becoming well again can go now.

These remaining feelings around not becoming well again have my permission to leave now.

These remaining feelings around not becoming well again feel like...

These remaining feelings around not becoming well again will not hold me back.

I am open to these remaining feelings leaving me now.

I am open to healing fully.

I am fully healed.

9. After another one or two rounds like this, see where the intensity of the issue is. If it's dropped again, you are on the right track; if it's down to zero, that's brilliant! If it's hardly budged at all, then you are still not working with the core issue of the problem.

10. Try another round of tapping if this is the case, using phrases like:

Even though I haven't got to the bottom of this issue, I am open to addressing it and know I will find a way to help myself.

I now let go of my attachments to these issues.

These feelings do not serve me; I let go of them now.

I thank my body and/or mind for protecting me, but they can let go of this now.

Even though I find this issue too upsetting to deal with right now, I know I am on the right track and I allow myself to be open and willing to heal.

If you haven't fully resolved your area of concern after tapping, don't worry about it; you have put some powerful tools in place, and your subconscious mind will be working its magic with them now. Give the tapping another go in a day or two and things may be different, and if they are not then tap on it not working, ask yourself how this makes you feel, and tap on those feelings. Either way, don't give yourself a hard time about it. If you are, then tap on that first as it will hold your healing back.

Use all your ailments, thoughts, and feelings as invitations from the body to resolve something else within you. Don't let them spiral out of control; tap on them as soon as you notice them, and use them to help you heal. They are there for a reason, and if you choose to listen you learn from them and will be able to move on. Even if you can't manage a whole tapping routine, do something, do anything, but just do it!

Visualising the health, harmony, and healing you want for yourself.

This next step to getting focused is an important yet very simple one. I'd like you to spend time every day visualising what you want from the program. This may be being fit, healthy, well, and thin (whatever the reason is for embarking on this cleanse, use it to visualise). This means instead of focusing every day on how unwell, unfit, or fat/thin you are, I would like to ask you to do the opposite. I don't mean think about how you want to be in the future; I mean focus on feeling that way now. When you look in the mirror, see yourself how you want to be. Start and/or finish all your meditations, quiet times, or even sleeps with a short visualisation where you fully embody being everything you are wanting to be now. Feel it, see it, love it, be it with every cell of your being.

When we are focusing on what we don't want every day, we are creating chemical reactions in the mind that reinforce these negative pathways and thus keep us unwell. However, when we spend time focusing on what we actually want (rather than how we feel we are right now), these same reactions happen but instead they create positive pathways for change, thus assisting the body to heal.

I can't state how incredibly powerful this simple technique is. It helped me so much with my own recovery from ME/CFS, and I know it helps so many others every single day. Make a pledge with yourself to try it for the duration of the cleanse, and see what a profound effect it can have on you.

Meditating your way to health and well-healing

The last tool I'm going to bestow on you for getting focused for this program is a simple meditation technique.

Even if you can only manage a short meditation every day, that's fine; anything is better than nothing at all. And for that reason, I'm going to assume that some readers may be new to meditating. If you've tried meditating before, you may have found it very difficult. To help, I've written some clear instructions below. You can also find a recording of this on my YouTube channel www.faithcanter.com/videos. You may find it useful to use it as a guided meditation.

Getting into a daily meditation practice will help reduce stress and anxiety, and many other health ailments both mental and physical, as it allows the body and mind to be in a harmonious healing state. It's also going to help the body repair itself.

1. Find a comfortable and supportive position to sit in (preferably, don't lie down unless you cannot manage to sit up, due to your health). Switch off phones and computers, or anything else that may distract you.

2. Breathe deeply and fully (making sure to expel all the stale air from your lungs, and bring in as much clean, refreshing air as possible) in through the nose and out through the mouth.

3. Now bring your awareness into the body as a whole (whilst continuing to breathe).

4. Allow your awareness to drift around the body until it comes to settle somewhere (this might not be where you expect, but just go with it). This could be an area you are aware of

(like a painful area), or it could be one where you are hold-ing stress or even where you are holding unwanted weight. The important thing is not to force your attention anywhere, but allow it to flow to the place it wants to.

5. Now, breathe in and out of this place, breathing in clean, cleansing, healing energy to this spot, and let go of stale, heavy, hindered energy and blockages with each out-breath. Allow your own breath to heal and cleanse this area for you.

6. Then breathe in love, breathe it into the whole area your awareness is in. Fully embody love within this area. When this area feels as cleansed and full of love as it wants to be for the time being, allow your awareness to take you to another place within your body (or even an energy field). Do the same cleansing breath and love work for this area as well.

7. Continue doing this until you feel your awareness has finished directing your healing energy around your body.

8. Bring your awareness into the full body. Take comfort in the fact you have allowed this wonderful, healing, and nurturing time for yourself, and thank yourself for this. I like to say thank you three times out loud, but do whatever works for you.

9. Slowly wiggle your fingers and toes, and open your eyes. You may wish to take another deep breath now and let go of any residual stale energy.

Hurdles to Healing

1. Why getting focused is so important. If you don't want this cleanse to feel like a burden, but to work and to last way past these six weeks, it's important you get focused for it by following the contents of the last chapter. I mean, do you want to find yourself doing yet another detox, diet, or program in another few months? No? I didn't think so.

2. What's holding you back from tapping/visualising/meditation? If you are finding the items in this chapter hard to get your head around, your day keeps getting away from you, or you are resisting them, then you may want to tap on these issues. Often there are resistances to change that we aren't even aware of and ignoring them won't work, so you may as well use them to help heal yourself. Symptoms, negative thoughts, and additional weight are all invitations for you to heal something in your life! Use them as the messages they are from your mind, and tap on these first.

3. Yes, you can meditate! Lots of people believe they can't meditate (I was one of those people). I'm here to tell you, you can! It's not about quietening the mind; it's about becoming the observer of your thoughts rather than being consumed by them. When you notice that you are thinking during meditation practice, simply honour the thoughts that are there and then let them go (like clouds leaving your vision), and then bring your attention back to your breath. Don't beat yourself up about thinking whilst mediating, it's perfectly normal. It's the beating yourself up that interferes with the meditation practice, and not the thought itself.

Reminder: Your tool-belt to health leading up to your cleanse is as follows:

1. Tapping/Emotional Freedom Technique (EFT)
2. Visualisation
3. Meditation

The more you do these, the better place your mind, body, and spirit will be for healing over the next six weeks.

Chapter 2: Get Purchased

As with all detox programs, there are some purchases to make. I hope that some of these things you'll already have hanging around, and many will last for several months after starting the detox program (so will form part of your new health habits going forward). And, of course, the perishables will nourish, nurture, and detox your system as part of this six-week program.

I have broken this chapter down into sections for you. There are purchases to be made for the fridge, for the larder, supplementation and equipment. These are just my suggestions based on my experience of taking other people through this program. There will, of course, be additional fresh produce to buy, depending on what meals you decide to eat from the recipes in the last section of this book. You can substitute items you don't like or would prefer not to purchase, but remember that we are aiming for health and wellbeing when you make your substitutes.

Please note there are two essential items in the supplement section that you will want to get ordered as soon as possible!

For the Fridge

Fresh ginger

Lemons and/or limes

Cucumber

Sweet potatoes

Red & white cabbages

Fresh garlic

Fresh oregano

Fresh parsley

Sauerkraut (raw)

Kimchi (raw)

Almond milk (homemade or unsweetened, if shop-bought)

A large selection of fresh vegetables

For the Larder

Various dried seaweeds (especially kombu/kelp)

Quinoa

Amaranth

Oats (gluten free)

Brown, black or red rice

Himalayan or sea salt

Flax seeds

Hemp seeds

Chia seeds

Olive oil (a good quality one)

Flax oil

Coconut oil (unrefined and organic)

Sesame seed oil

Tahini

Dried ginger

Dandelion and/or nettle tea bags (unbleached and organic)

Dried wormwood

Dried walnut leaf

Dried cloves

Supplementation

Grapefruit seed extract (not to be confused with grape seed oil) - ESSENTIAL

Oregano oil - ESSENTIAL

B12 subliminal (as a lozenge, spray or drops)

Magnesium (as a lozenge, spray, drops or homeopathic remedy)

Zinc (as a lozenge, spray, drops or homeopathic remedy)

Raw protein powder (I like the Sunwarrior brand)

Zeolites (liquid clay)

Equipment

Rebounder (mini trampoline)

Zapper (optional)

A BPA free water filter

Soft body brush (although you can just use your hands)

Smoothie maker (or blender of some description)

Chapter 3: Get Prepared

During this program, you will be cleansing mind, body, and home, to allow you to live in health, harmony, and happiness. It's important that you understand why you might not already be living in health and harmony, and how this program is going to help.

Most of us have had times in our lives where we have burnt the candle at both ends (or maybe we still are), where we've had a poor diet, been on antibiotics, oral contraceptives, steroids, drunk too much, dieted too hard, become stressed and anxious too often, been through traumatic events, or a combination of these. Any one of these items by itself can cause health problems, but when we add a few of them together over a prolonged period, our body and mind become out of balance and work in a far less harmonious and nurturing way. This slowly but surely can lead to a whole host of health concerns, both mental and physical. Quite often you might go to see someone at this stage, you might be prescribed something, or try a new treatment or therapy, and you may or may not feel a little better for a while. But then either the same issue rears its head or another similar one does. You see, unless we can learn to live in harmony with body and mind then we are just borrowing from Peter to pay Paul. What *Cleanse* does is to get back to basics, to clear and cleanse the body and mind through a process of life detoxification, but in a nurturing and healing way. It focuses on reducing toxins coming into body and mind, and assisting your body to let go of the ones already on board.

As such, it's important to prepare yourself for the six weeks ahead to make the most of the program and benefit from it fully. You can do this by...

1. Setting aside six weeks where you don't have lots of parties, you aren't travelling or attending lots of social events.

2. Use up all processed foods, especially anything with sugar and gluten in it.

3. Use up all natural sugars, including fruits and things like honey (the reasons for this will be explained later).

4. Buying as much of the 'get purchased' items as possible.

5. Read through the recipes in the back of this book and pick the ones that you like the sound of.

6. Make a shopping list with the things you need, after picking the recipes you like from the back of the book.

7. Plan some time in your diary each day for the parts of the book that will help you nourish and nurture your mind.

8. If you are doing this program for weight loss, weigh yourself now – then not again until the end.

9. Get others onboard, as it's always easier when doing any sort of program with other people (especially partners or family members you live with), or even start up a Facebook or WhatsApp Group and support each other.

10. Use the 'getting focused' chapter to help you do just that.

The list below contains some ways that you can support your body through this program. These are simple items that can be added in before even starting the full detox, and continued after the program has finished. If you start some of these now they will assist your body and mind to eliminate toxins more effectively and help to minimise detox symptoms.

1. Reduce the toxic load in your food. Start replacing processed foods with healthier options.

2. Reduce your use of sugars, sweeteners, diet foods and drinks, caffeine and alcohol.

3. Think about the toxic load of your cosmetics and hair care products (we absorb around 60% of what we put onto our bodies). Consider replacing these with natural, organic versions when they run out. Or even consider making your own if you'd like to save money and the environment as well. My book *Living a Life Less Toxic* has many simple recipes for doing this.

4. Think about the toxic load of your cleaning products, and consider replacing them with more natural options when they run out. If it touches your skin, it's likely you are absorbing it, and if it's smelly then you are breathing it into those beautiful lungs. There's not much that vinegar and bicarbonate of soda can't clean in a house, and not only is this super cheap, but it means that less toxins are being absorbed by your body. Again, my book *Living a Life Less Toxic* has lots of cheap and easy recipes for making your own.

5. Drink plenty of water (at least 2-3 litres every day, and more if exercising). Try to drink from a non-plastic, or at least a BPA-free plastic, container. This will help your lymphatic system eliminate toxins. Preferably drink at least a litre of water as soon as you wake up, and before doing anything else with your day.

6. Consider doing some simple exercise regularly. This doesn't need to be high impact – just a minimum of 20 minutes, four times a week. This helps your body sweat out toxins.

7. Consider investing in a good probiotic (with many billion and multi-strain live bacteria in it).

8. Invest in some bitter teas; dandelion and nettle are ideal. The more bitter the better for helping the liver with detoxification.

9. Increase your consumption of magnesium-rich foods (leafy greens, nuts, seeds, beans, lentils, fish, avocados, figs, bananas, and whole grains).

10. Try to have as many Epsom salt baths as possible. Epsom salts are high in magnesium and help to draw out toxins and assist with so many areas of health. Add at least 3 mugs of salts to a bath, and soak for a minimum of 20 minutes.

11. Consider regular massage, reflexology, saunas, steam rooms or any other detoxifying therapies. These therapies stimulate the lymphatics, helping them to eliminate toxins through our skin and via our urine.

12. Take up body brushing. You can use a long-handled brush or just your own hands, and brush your skin towards the area

just about your breasts. Make sure that you brush up the sides of your breasts (even for men), as a lot of toxins are stored in breast tissue. Your breasts may become tender, but this will pass. Body brushing removes blockages in the lymphatic system, and helps this system to eliminate toxins more effectively. I can't emphasise enough how good body brushing is for you. Even if you are not ready to do anything else at all from this book, starting to body brush daily will have a huge impact on your toxic load.

13. Make sure you are having at least one bowel movement each day. Bowel movements are one of the body's main ways to remove toxins. If you're not having regular bowel movements, try eating more fibre, drinking more water, and take up body brushing and rebounding.

14. Try daily rebounding (jumping on a mini trampoline), as this helps stimulate the lymphatics.

15. Reduce your use of, or eliminate antiperspirants. These products impair the body's ability to eliminate toxins through sweating. Bad body odour is caused by toxins leaving the body, so this will pass once you have eliminated these toxins.

16. Try to get a minimum of eight hours' sleep a night. Your body does a lot of its detoxing during the night!

17. If you don't understand the ingredients list in a food, avoid it. Strange words on labels usually mean chemicals!

18. Try some regular deep breathing. Breathe deeply and fully into the lungs, stomach and back. This will help your body remove toxins from the respiratory system, and allow the

rest of your body to get the energy and oxygen it requires to do its job effectively.

19. Get out and connected with nature more! Why? Check out below...

When we connect regularly with nature, we disperse the effects of electromagnetic stress. We and the planet vibrate at a negative frequency, whereas electrical appliances vibrate at a positive frequency. In the past, our relationship with our planet was different: we slept on the land; we worked it; and it provided our food and drink. We no longer do much of this today. We actually spend very little time in contact with nature, and yet we wonder why we feel so out of sync and poorly so much of the time. Being constantly surrounded by electromagnetic fields (EMF) and deprived of nature interferes with our immune, nervous, and endocrine systems, and can also create symptoms like:

− Colds, flu, and general ill health

− Anxiety, depression, aggression, irritability

− Insomnia and general sleep problems

− Memory loss and brain fog

− Increased chance of (particularly epileptic) seizures

− Dizziness, vertigo, disorientation

− Fatigue

− Respiratory issues

− Loss of appetite, over-eating and nausea

− High blood pressure and haemorrhage

- Issues with the eyes in general, but particularly in the cornea and dry/itchy eyes and poor vision

- Eczema, dry, itchy skin, dermatitis, and allergies

- Joint and muscle pain

- Tinnitus and other hearing difficulties

- Persistent detox symptoms, burning sensations, and sweating

- Shaking and jitters

- Developmental issues in children and adults alike

- Not feeling grounded

The good news is that we can make some simple changes to reduce these symptoms:

1. Unplug yourself. By this I mean spend some time away from all appliances, in the garden, on a walk or at the beach, away from as many electrical appliances as possible.

2. Remove as many electrical appliances from your bedroom as possible. Especially anything that is receiving or emitting signals of any sort.

3. Ditch the electric blanket; these are possibly one of the worst items for increasing electromagnetic stress, because they are so close to us for so many hours at a time.

4. Switch off as many appliances at night as possible, and whenever you are not using them.

5. Do away with your microwave. Not only do microwaves

break down most of the nutrients in your food, they are also a big source of electromagnetic stress.

6. Cordless phones are just as bad as mobile phones, so if you need to use these, then try storing them as far away from your body as possible when not in use.

7. Purchase a grounding mat or blanket for your bed. When you are sleeping, you will be grounding yourself. These earth through the normal plug sockets in your home.

8. Practise grounding meditations and visualisations.

9. Consider wearing and/or placing any of the following crystals next to you, your bed, or desk, to help minimise the effects of electromagnetic stress: Smoky quartz, Hematite, Tourmalated quartz, Black tourmaline, Amazonite, Sodalite, and Unakite.

10. Purchase a bio-band, a bio-tag, a grounding egg, earthing necklace, or one of the other many grounding items you can carry around on your person all the time to help deflect the harmful effects of electromagnetic stress.

11. Drink plenty of fresh, pure water as this has a wonderful grounding effect on the body.

12. Use a Zapper. These not only help with many different areas of health (like detoxing from heavy metals and parasites, etc), but they also help with grounding. This is because they emit a very low dose of negatively charged electricity, much the same as when the body is in contact with the planet.

13. Ground/earth yourself. By this I mean go outside barefoot, with as much skin as possible touching the earth, and spend some time connected with nature. Connecting with the earth rebalances the body and brings us back to its natural rhythm and function. Paddling in the sea, hugging a tree (yes, hugging a tree), or gardening without gloves: all these are just as effective as wandering around barefoot for a while. This is particularly helpful before and after flying to prevent jet-lag.

As you can see, there are many things that you can do prior to, during, and after your cleanse to assist your body and mind to let go, clear out, and heal. Pick the things that resonate with you the most and start there.

Hurdles to Healing

1. The more you do prior to the cleanse the less the detox symptoms will affect you during the program. You don't want to be giving up because you feel so rubbish a few weeks down the line, so I highly recommend you try to do some of the things outlined in this chapter prior to starting the program.

2. Some of the simplest things, like getting outside more, can have such a profound effect on health. Just because it seems simple it doesn't mean it's not powerful, so don't be fooled by this!

3. Get others on board with the program (if not all of it, then some of it). When other people around you are enjoying

some of the 'toxic luxuries' that you can't, it can make staying on the program much harder. See if there is anyone that will do this with you, and then support each other.

4. And remember – keep tapping on anything and everything that is bothering you, as it is bothering you. It's your body speaking to you and asking for you to resolve what has manifested.

Section Two:
The Cleanse Program

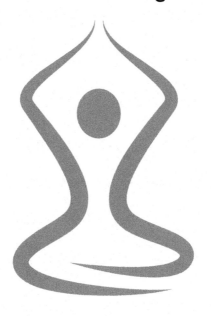

Chapter 4: Week One

Now that you are prepared and focused, it's time to start the program. Week one is all about things that you can add to your daily regime, rather than taking away. This will support your body through this holistic detox program and ensure you are getting the nutrients you require.

It's important to focus firstly on what we can add. This ensures we are getting everything we need and, thus, our body and mind aren't in starvation mode. When we are in starvation mode we hold onto things, both mentally and physically. These things include what we are eating (so it can actually make us fat) and also attachments to people, events and places that we need to let go of. Spending the first week adding rather than removing too much, helps to ensure that our body and mind don't go into panic mode and that we are doing all we can to minimize any detox symptoms.

So, let's fill up and let go this week!

Letting Go with Tapping:

1. Think of times, people, places or ailments in your life that you may be holding on to. Which one is bothering you the most, which one do you feel is unresolved or that triggers something in you when you think of it? Now think of the first time this occurred, and rate this feeling out of ten.

2. Start by saying the set-up phrase: 'Even though I am holding onto that which does not serve me, I deeply and completely love and accept myself.' If you struggle to say this, then try opting for one of the other set-up phrases in the 'Getting Focused' chapter earlier in the book; or, better still, work on what's holding you back from saying this first.

3. Whilst saying this set-up phrase three times, tap the top of your head (see the 'Getting Focused' chapter for exact tapping points).

4. Now move on to tapping the other points in turn, as explained previously. Say out loud how you felt at the time, about whatever it is you feel that you've been holding on to. Use as much detail, emotions, and even physical feelings as you can. Get it all out, no matter how irrelevant it may seem. Keep going, moving onto each new tapping point until you feel everything is out.

5. Now take a few deep breaths and rate the feelings out of ten. If the number has not moved down to a zero, then there is still some work to be done. If it has gone down by a few numbers, then we are on the right track. If it has not gone down at all, you may be tapping on something other than the core concern for you. If this is the case, see if there's another event prior to this one which made you feel the same or similar way, and work on that instead.

6. The next round of tapping works in exactly the same way, but start adding in phrases like:

I'm open to healing from this.

I give myself permission to fully heal from this.

I let go of these thoughts and feelings that no longer serve me.

I know I can fully heal and move on from this.

I let go of...

I'm no longer holding on to this...

I am prepared to make changes in my life that nourish me more.

I'm making changes that nurture me more.

I'm worth it.

7. Keep going until you feel you have got everything out, and then take a few deep breaths and assess how you feel about the situation now. If it's not gone down to zero but has moved down, then keep going, adding in anything you feel could be holding you back or that is upsetting you about the situation. If it is down to zero, then move on to any other things you feel you are still holding onto that may not be serving you.

Healing with Visualisation

Start and/or finish all your meditations, quiet times or even sleeps, with a short visualisation where you fully embody being everything you want to be: feel it, see it, be it, love it! Be it with every cell of your being. Imagine your body literally letting go of that which does not serve it, lightening its load, healing and becoming more harmonious.

Letting Go with Meditation

1. Find a comfortable and supportive position to sit in (preferably, don't lie down unless you cannot manage sitting). Switch off phones and computers or anything else that may distract you.

2. Breathe deeply and fully (making sure to expel all the stale air from your lungs and bring in as much clean, refreshing air as possible) in through the nose and out through the mouth.

3. Now bring your awareness into the body as a whole (whilst continuing to breathe).

4. Imagine a bright cleansing light coming down from above, entering your head, clearing out and replacing all the stale, negative thoughts, habits, and programs.

5. Allow this bright cleansing light to slowly make its way down through the rest of your head, cleaning and clearing as it goes, removing stress, pain, illness, and tension as it moves down towards your neck and throat.

6. As it enters your throat, know that it is clearing any blockages here, allowing you to speak your truth. Let go of any words you regret saying and any that you did not say but wish you had. Know that the light is allowing you to forgive yourself and others as it works its way down to your shoulders.

7. Know that the healing light is literally allowing you to lighten your load here, allowing you to put down all those things

you have been carrying (of your own and of other people's). Feel the stress and tension leave your shoulders, and know that by letting go of these burdens you are doing yourself and others a great service.

8. Now the bright healing light enters your chest and upper back. Feel it opening up this area, making its way into the dark, closed, and uncomfortable places. Brightening and lightening as it goes, allowing you to let go of tension and allowing your lungs to fill full of cleansing and nurturing air, healing your heartaches and your sadness. Allowing you to cut cords to other people's heartache and sadness as well. Feel your own energy returning to you and all parts of you that may have been attached to others, now making you whole.

9. The light moves down into the middle of your body, healing, cleansing, and cleaning as it makes its way down through your digestive system. Healing you from the inside out, removing blockages and stale energies.

10. As the light enters your hips and then your upper legs, know that you are letting go of anything preventing you from moving forward, from healing, and from anything preventing you from nourishing yourself.

11. The bright healing light is now making its way down through your legs. Feel it removing that stale energy, fatigue, and anything making you feel stuck or trapped.

12. The healing light is now moving into your ankles and feet, where it allows you to feel grounded and connected to all, like you never have before. You are fully supported in this

process, and you are just where you need to be to begin moving forward with a new, nourishing and healing part of your journey.

13. The healing light is now moving through you and into the ground, where it is connecting you to the earth, to Mother Nature, and to life as a whole.

14. You are now completely full of this healing light. It's allowing you to let go, move on, and connect to who you really are. Feel the connection to the earth, take this with you through-out your day. You are loved and nurtured now and every day.

15. Bring your awareness into the full body, take comfort in the fact you have allowed this wonderful, healing and nurturing time for yourself, and thank yourself for this. I like to say thank you three times out loud, but do whatever feels right for you.

16. Slowly wiggle your fingers and toes and open your eyes. You may wish to take another deep breath now and let go of any residual stale energy.

17. Repeat this meditation technique at least once a day.

The body detox bit

When we heal the digestive system, the rest of the body will follow suit as it supports most functions within the body. Good digestive health is fundamental to a well-functioning body, and here are some of the reasons why:

1. With a fully functioning digestive system, toxicity of the body will be greatly reduced: the digestive system will be able to eliminate more of the toxins from food and drink consumed. A balance of good and bad bacteria in the digestive system will be achieved. When the bad bacteria get out of hand, they create more toxins as they grow, raising the body's toxicity levels.

2. Many digestive-based illnesses like IBS and food intolerances completely heal when you take time to heal this system of the body.

3. Your digestive enzyme levels will be higher, enabling the body to process foods and absorb nutrients from your food.

4. Most of your immune system is based in your digestive system, so when you heal the digestive system you'll also heal your immune system.

5. Most of the serotine (one of our happy hormones), is produced in the digestive system. Thus, a happy digestive system often means a happy head.

6. Inflammation in the body will be greatly reduced, which helps a whole host of other health complaints, including arthritis, joint, and muscular pain.

7. If you are looking to improve your memory, have better mental clarity, or even sleep better, then these can all be significantly improved through healing the digestive system.

8. If the body isn't using lots of energy trying to process foods and drinks that it's struggling with, then that energy becomes available to you for day-to-day things instead.

This means that by healing the digestive system, you'll also increase your energy and vitality for life.

Starting the process of healing the digestive system is quite simple. We can do this by adding in some simple foods and drinks to help nurture the ecology of the digestive system, and that also gives us more of the nutrients we require for repairing, replenishing, and strengthening the body.

In my opinion, one of the best things we can add into our diet for digestive health and general wellbeing is fermented foods and drinks.

Fermented foods encourage good gut health. By fermented food, I don't mean pickled foods, as these have a minimal amount of goodness left in them. By fermented, I mean cultured (food and drink traditionally made with a cultured starter), or lacto-fermented (traditionally made with salt and water). Both processes are highly nutritious and also help you to absorb the nutrients from other foods and drinks. They are full of millions of beneficial yeasts and bacteria and are wonderfully detoxifying for the digestive system. They also help to address any imbalance of good and bad yeasts within the body. Different types of fermented foods have slightly different strains of probiotics, so having a good range of these foods prepared in different ways is highly beneficial to your body. They can all be prepared at home very cheaply and easily, or you can buy most of them from any good health food shop, or even online. When purchasing them, make sure they are unpasteurised, so they are still full of all the health benefits that pasteurised options often lack. For the next few weeks, please do not consume kombucha or water kefir (two of the fermented drinks), because unless you know what you are doing you may find they still have too much sugar, or the other way, have become a bit alcoholic to consume during the cleanse program.

There's lots of fermented vegetable recipes in the back of this book that you can choose from. I highly recommend the sauerkraut or the kimchi to start with, as they are super simple to make and very yummy! Start with a small amount (maybe a teaspoon's worth) and slowly build up, otherwise you may find the detox symptoms are a lot stronger than you would like. And if you do find this is the case, then simply take a little less the next time.

Seaweed

Seaweed is highly nutritious, easily absorbable, and we simply don't eat enough of it these days. Different seaweeds have slightly different nutritional contents, so having a good selection of them in your diet is a great idea. Seaweed has a high protein content as well as being high in calcium, iodine, magnesium, and vitamin B and C. It also helps blood sugar levels, liver function, brain health, thyroid health, diabetes, is anti-bacterial, anti-inflammatory, and anti-viral, and assists the body with detoxing. You can get more nutrients from a single serving of seaweed than from many other things you eat day-to-day. What's more, it's super easy to get more of this wonder food into your diet. Even if you don't like the taste of seaweed, you can use one of the many organic seaweed shakers you can pick up in health food stores or online to sprinkle some seaweed into most meals, in a way you don't taste.

A little seaweed and some sesame seed oil makes a great and healthy alternative to soya sauce in any dish, hot or cold.

Start adding this nutrient dense food into your diet today, to improve the level of nutrients you are consuming right from the beginning of this holistic detox program, and keep adding it way into the future, too.

Smoothies

Dust off the smoothie maker and check out all the healthy, yet yummy smoothie recipes in the back of this book. Start today with adding in at least one green smoothie a day. Smoothies are a great way to get a lot of nutrients into our diet in one go. Keeping them as green as possible helps balance the blood sugar levels (too much fruit sugar may counteract this, which is also the reason we won't be juicing during the cleanse program).

The more nutrients you get into the body, the better it will function, the healthier it will be, the more energy you will have, and believe it or not, the more likely it is you'll lose weight.

Check out the recipes, make a shopping list, and get supping!

Supplements

As a general rule of thumb, if your digestive system isn't working as effectively as it should be, then you won't be absorbing the nutrients you require from the food and drink you consume. If you clean up the digestive system and eat a good balanced diet, then you'll more than likely get what you need from what you consume.

If you feel your digestive system needs cleaning up, you could be deficient in something and are not likely to be getting it from your diet. I recommend that you invest in a good quality supplement in a drop, patch, lozenge or spray, as these won't rely on the digestive system for absorption.

There are a few supplements which I feel are beneficial to detoxing, health, and healing. These are:

Magnesium: Most people I come across are magnesium deficient. Magnesium helps the body to detox, soothes the sympathetic nervous system, and helps aid sleep (which is when we do much of our detoxing). Epsom salt baths are a great way to draw out toxins and put in magnesium. Try having several of these a week over the next few weeks, or at least foot baths with them in if you don't have a bath. Add at least three mugs of salts to each bath, and try to sit in it for at least 20 minutes.

B12: This vitamin is essential to good health, both mentally and physically, and is very hard to absorb enough of naturally. It helps with energy levels, mental function, mood, and digestive function. It also assists against stroke, cholesterol, high blood pressure, and Alzheimer's. I recommend a Methylcobalamin B12.

Zinc: Many people are deficient in zinc. Zinc is a great antioxidant, helps us sleep, and increases energy levels, as well as aiding the immune system and a whole host of other things throughout the body.

Zeolites (liquid clay): Clays are a great way to assist the body with detoxing. Liquid clays, unlike many other clays, are easier to use and consume. Zeolite clay re-mineralises the body, supports the immune system, rebalances the pH level of the body, increases serotine in the body, and removes many toxins, including heavy metals.

That's a Wrap for Week One

As you can see, we are adding in lots of lovely, healthy goodness, and the only things I am going to recommend you remove at this stage is alcohol, processed sugars, and processed meals in general. Start having a look through the recipes in the back of this book, see what you like the sound of, and maybe try out one or two. When you find any recipes you like, I recommend that you make more than you need and freeze the rest for those nights when you want something easy, yet healthy, to eat.

The more nourishing choices you make for yourself now, the easier any detox symptoms will be for you during the rest of the cleanse.

You'll find a nourishment chart at the end of each of the next few chapters of the cleanse program. Each chart is designed to help you keep track of what I recommend for cleansing, nourishing, and nurturing body and mind during each week of this holistic detox program.

You can photocopy each chart if you wish, or use it within the book. Tick off each thing as you do it each day, and it will remind you what to do when.

NOURISHMENT CHART - WEEK ONE							
	M	T	W	T	F	S	S
Morning							
Meditate (or do this whenever it feels right)							
Visualise							
Body Brushing (after bath or shower)							
Green Smoothie							
Drink 2-3 ltrs of water (throughout the day)							
Zinc							
Magnesium							
Zeolite Clay							
B12							
Afternoon							
Visualise							
Reduce Caffeine							
Make a nourishing lunch choice							
Fermented Veggies							
Evening							
Tapping (or do this whenever it feels right)							
Visualise							
Make a nourishing dinner choice							
Fermented Veggies							
Add some Seaweed to dinner (or lunch)							
Epsom salt bath							
No processed meals							
No processed sugars							
No alcohol							

Hurdles to Healing

1. Get everything ordered before you put this book down, then nothing gets in the way.

2. Try to get a friend to do the cleanse with you; you can support each other.

3. Remind yourself why you are doing this, and journal if you find it helpful.

4. Tap on whatever is holding you back, or whatever you have reservations about.

Chapter 5: Week Two

This week we concentrate on swapping out some of the naughty foods and drinks for not-so-naughty ones. We will also be continuing to support you with nurturing meditations, tapping routines, and visualisations.

Let's start with a simple tapping routine that will gear you up for the next few weeks. We often don't take the time to thank our bodies for everything they are doing for us each and every day. In fact, instead of being grateful for our bodies, we more often than not are doing the complete opposite and finding fault, due to health concerns or image issues. For this reason, during this week's mind detox sessions we'll be focusing on gratitude for our body. Each day our body gets us up and moving, it takes us from A to B, it pumps blood and nutrients around itself, and protects us from the elements, as well as from ourselves when we are not in a nurturing state of mind. It's really extraordinary how many millions of things happen in our body every second of every day. So, let's big-up-the-body this week and give it the gratitude it deserves. Focusing on gratitude for the body will create more things to be grateful for. When we focus on the negative, that's where our energy goes; we reinforce those negative pathways within the brain that create chemical reactions to reinforce those thoughts. But when we focus on the positive, we reinforce those positive pathways within the brain, creating positive chemical reactions that nurture health rather than hinder it.

Gratitude Tapping

1. Start by saying the set-up phrase: 'Even though my body doesn't always do what I want it to do, I deeply love and accept myself.' If you struggle to say this, then try opting for one of the other set-up phrases in the 'Getting Focused' chapter earlier in the book; or, better still, work on what's holding you back from saying this first.

2. Whilst saying this set-up phrase three times, tap the top of your head (see the 'Getting Focused' chapter for exact tapping points).

3. Now move on to tapping the other points in turn, as explained previously. Say out loud how you feel about your body, that means all the nasty things you usually only say within your head. Get them all out whilst you tap, this will help you use them to heal and break down blockages and habits based on them. Get it all out, no matter how irrelevant it may seem. Keep going, moving onto each new tapping point until you feel everything is out.

4. Now it's time to start tapping on what you like about your body or what you are grateful for. This could be things like your lips, your hearing, your hair, how your body gets you from A to B, how it pumps blood around itself, how it works without you having to do anything.

5. Once you have tapped through every tiny thing you can think of to be grateful to your body for, start tapping on the following.

   Thank you, body, for always doing what's best for me, even when it doesn't feel that way to me.

   Thank you, body, for protecting me, even when it doesn't feel to me like you are doing this. I know you only have my best interests at heart.

   Thank you, body, for all the amazing things you do for me each and every day.

   Thank you for waking up every day.

   I am sorry I have not treated you as well as I should.

   I am sorry I've seen you as separate to me; I understand now we are connected, and I embrace that connection.

   Thank you for your support, your protection, and your nurturing nature.

   Thank you for all you do for me, but when you wish to help and protect me now and in the future, can you do it in not such a painful or uncomfortable way?

   I promise to listen when you speak and not ignore your messages.

   Thank you, thank you, thank you for all you do each and every day.

6. Keep going until you feel you have got everything out. If you have been bad to your body in any way, then make sure

to apologise to it now for that and to be grateful for the messages it was trying to tell you.

7. When you are completely done, take a few deep breaths, breathing out any residual negativity towards your body and breathing in gratitude and thanks for all it has, is, and will do for you.

Cleansing with Visualisation

Start and/or finish all your meditations, quiet times, or even sleeps, with a short visualisation where you fully embody being everything you are wanting to be now. Feel it, see it, be it, love it! Be it with every cell of your being.

Visualise yourself walking towards a stream or small river within a beautiful healing valley. As you get closer, you can feel the power of the water. You know this is exactly what you require at this time. Sit down next to the flowing water and touch it. You are surprised how warm it is, so much so that you find yourself getting slowly into the water. As you slide into the water, you can feel all that heaviness, all that negativity about your body, and all those aches and pains, literally being washed away. Take some deep breaths and let out any residual negativity that may be hiding deep within. Let it all go. Let the water cleanse you of all that does not serve you presently. As you let go, you feel your muscles relaxing, you feel nature nurturing you, and you are grateful for what passed before as it has led you to this place, to this healing, and to this moment. When you feel completely cleansed by the water, slowly make your way back to the bank and lay out on the green grass, in the warm sun, and dry off in perfect peace. Ground yourself now with the earth as you dry off and rest fully within your body. Love your body for all it has done and all it will do. Now, slowly, come back to the present moment within the room you are in, but bring that pure, cleansing feeling of the water and that place in nature with you.

Cleansing with Meditation

1. Find a comfortable and supportive position to sit in (preferably don't lie down unless you cannot manage to sit up due to your health). Switch off phones, computers, and anything else that may distract you.

2. Breathe deeply and fully (making sure to expel all the stale air from your lungs, and bring in as much clean refreshing air as possible) in through the nose and out through the mouth.

3. Now bring your awareness to your heart centre, and imagine a light pink cleansing light within your heart centre, one that is very slowly growing.

4. The ball of light pink light is expanding slowly, out through your heart and into the rest of the chest, front and back.

5. It is now filling your torso and moving further outwards into all other areas of your body, filling up any uncomfortable, painful, or displeasing areas of your body. When you come across these areas, make sure to fully allow the pink light to engulf them.

6. The light pink cleansing light now fills your whole body and is spilling out into the area you occupy within the room, then within the building you are in, and the street, the town, and the county you are in.

7. The light pink cleansing light continues to spill out of you, overflowing into the country you are in, and then the continent and then the whole world.

8. It doesn't stop here, though. This light pink light flows out into the universe; cleansing, healing, and purifying all there is.

9. Stay with this for a while, being fully aware of the area this light pink cleansing light now covers.

10. Slowly roll back in the light pink light, slowly bringing it back to the planet, to the continent, the country, county, town, street, building, and room.

11. Now bring the light back into your body and just rest for a moment in the perfection that you are, that life is, and take comfort in the fact you have allowed this wonderful, healing, and nurturing time for yourself, and thank yourself for this. I like to say thank you three times out loud, but do whatever works for you.

12. Slowly wiggle your fingers and toes and open your eyes, but bring that pink cleansing light with you into your day-to-day activities. You may wish to take another deep breath now and let go of any residual stale energy.

13. Repeat this meditation technique at least once a day, but preferably twice.

The body detox bit

This week we are focused on what good things we can swap for not-so-good things. This way you shouldn't feel deprived in any way, and these should be nice easy swaps you can continue with after this six-week cleanse has finished. These swaps will ensure you get the nourishment your body requires, as well as stabilising your blood sugar (thus your mood, energy, and hormones as well). These foods will also stop you feeding the bad yeasts and parasites (more about this later) within your body.

The idea from this week onwards is that you try swapping out all the items below. This will make the cleanse easier in the following weeks (which is when we start healing the digestive system and, thus, the rest of the body).

I know it can seem confusing when trying to pick healthier options, as there are so many conflicting articles and research out there about foods and drinks. For instance, Wednesday's article says to drink coffee as it's full of antioxidants, yet Thursday's article says to not drink coffee as it's bad for your hormones. So, which one do you believe?

Here's a great rule of thumb which shouldn't serve you wrong... Consume foods and drinks as close to their nature state of growth as possible. What I mean by this is that if they have been overly processed to a state where they do not look anything like they did when they came off the plant or animal, then the chances are they aren't very good for you. So, pick chocolate without lots of added naughty things, such as dark natural chocolate, or even better raw. Eat bread that has naturally risen and not been forced; eat organic where possible, or grow your own. Eat food and drinks that resemble the items they are and not pre-packed with added naughty things. There is generally a raw, fermented, or healthy version of most things out there. But don't get caught out by the items calling themselves natural, organic, sugar, fat or wheat-free. Many apparent health foods are free from one naughty, only to be full of lots of others (especially sugar in the free-from section). This is why I say to pick the items that resemble their natural state the most, and don't get sucked in by the 'healthy' option labels. The fact that they still have tons of ingredients on the label suggests they are not what they may seem.

Ask yourself:

— Does this item resemble its natural state?

— Does it have lots of added ingredients?

— Do I know what these added ingredients are?

— Then lastly, ask yourself, is this item going to nourish my mind, body, or soul?

You'll soon have your answer if you want to buy and consume this item, without having to consult a food scientist!

Become a conscious food shopper/eater, instead of unconsciously throwing things in the basket in the vain hope they'll turn your health around because you read an article that proclaimed this magical food would help you lose weight, or reduce your arthritis, or whatever the article suggested. Instead, consider if this food is as close to its natural state as possible. Natural means nurturing; it means the body finds it easier to absorb the goodness from the food, to process the food, and to use what is within the food to be used by the body. If there are any chemical components in the food, then the body will not recognise these. And if it does not recognise something it consumes, then it may not be able to eliminate it, and may store it instead. This is when we get a build-up of chemicals, the body's toxic load rises, and health issues start to crop up. For those struggling to lose weight, you may wish to know that when the body stores these chemicals, it more often than not stores them in fat cells around our middle. This means that by reducing the chemicals we consume alone, we can actually lose weight, especially around our middles.

So, this week let's swap out the naughty for the not-so-naughty, but also remember to be a conscious consumer moving forward, and to pick natural-looking foods over 'healthy' or 'low fat/sugar/calorie' etc.

White rice – Brown Rice or Quinoa

White rice (like most of the white carbs and foods high on the GI index) helps to spike our blood sugar levels, thus interfering with our mood, energy levels, hormones, and feeds the bad yeasts within the digestive system. Swapping white rice for a slow releasing carb will not only give you a more balanced release of energy, but will assist in balancing all the above-mentioned systems of the body. If you don't like brown rice or can't be bothered waiting the extra time it takes to cook it, then try black or red rice, and know that you can buy many of them precooked these days. I personally like to batch cook mine, then freeze it down into portion sizes and take out just what I need, when I need it.

Couscous – Quinoa

A lot of people have moved over to couscous, thinking it's a healthy option. However, if you are trying to go wheat-free, I'm sorry to tell you it's not for you. Opt for quinoa instead, and you won't regret it. It can be purchased everywhere these days, even precooked and packaged, if that takes your fancy. It can be eaten hot with meals instead of rice, as a porridge or cereal, and also cold in salads, etc. For the vegetarians out there, it's also a great source of protein and carbohydrates. It also helps to clean the sides of the digestive system as it works its way through. It's a super little superfood indeed!

White Processed Sugars and Sweeteners – Honey (preferably raw)

When something says it's sugar-free, please don't assume this means healthy, as more often than not this means packed full of chemical sweeteners that the body will store instead, or eliminate. The best option is to sweeten foods yourself with natural sweeteners. Honey, in my opinion, is the best option, especially a raw honey as it not only sweetens your food and drink but it also gives you a wonderful supply of nutrients. Raw is always best as it's also packed full of lots of enzymes, but if you are going to be heating it then a standard honey is fine. Other natural sweeteners are things like agave nectar and maple syrup. Just be aware of how much of these you are having, though, because even the natural stuff, if consumed to excess, will spike your blood sugars eventually. Moderation is the best policy here!

White Flours – Wholemeal Flours (or gluten-free flours)

As with the white rice above, white flours spike the blood sugar levels, thus upsetting the same areas of the body and mind that white rice does. So, if you can't bear to be without your toast in the morning, the best option is to swap the white bread for wholemeal, which won't spike your blood sugars in quite the same way.

Bread – Sourdough

Whilst we are on the subject of bread, let's discuss sourdough. Sourdough is a great bready option, especially if it's sourdough you have made yourself or that has been more traditionally made. This is because it will have been allowed to rise naturally and not forced with yeasts, like many shop-purchased breads. This means it's not had naughty ingredients added to it, and will also have less, or even no gluten (depending on the sourdough). It's heavier bread because it's naturally risen, but it's a much better bread for you, and much closer to how we would have made bread many years ago.

White Potatoes – Sweet Potatoes

Once again, we are swapping a white carb for a slow-releasing and healthier carb. Not only will sweet potatoes not spike your blood sugars in the same way as white potatoes, but they are also jam-packed full of goodness. They can also be eaten raw as a pasta substitute (when put through a spiraliser). And sweet potato wedges allow you to feel that you can still have some comfort food.

Margarine – Organic Butter

Unfortunately, even though we have had many years of being told margarines are better for us than butters, we are now realising this is simply not true. Margarines are generally processed trans-fats, and as such they are not very recognisable to our bodies. Our bodies store them in our fat cells, thus making us fatter rather than thinner, as was initially thought when these fats were first produced. Butters are less processed, so the body can absorb and digest them in a natural and healthy way. Unfortunately, many dairy items these days have added hormones, antibiotics, and other chemicals added into that food chain at source, as these are what many dairy cows are given. So, organic butter and dairy, in general, is a much better option for overall health and weight loss.

Sunflower and Vegetable Oils – Coconut or Olive Oil

Sunflower and vegetable oils are also trans-fats. The body cannot process these items normally, as it does not recognise them, so it stores them in our cells, which then leads to a whole host of health complaints. Where possible, it's best to avoid items cooked in, or containing, trans-fats. Coconut oil is an amazing fat to cook with. It's the only oil that retains its nutritional content when heated to high temperatures and, boy, does it ever have a high nutritional content! A good quality olive oil is great for lower temperatures and salad dressing, etc, and sesame seed oil makes a great salad or stir-fry dressing (especially with a bit of seaweed – making a great alternative to soya sauce as well).

Monosodium Glutamate (MSG) – Just about any other herb or spice

MSG is a flavour enhancer which also makes you feel very full-up one moment and then starving again the next. It's found in most processed foods and a lot of takeaways. It's not a very nice 'food' item. So much so, it's a bit like a slow-releasing mild poison on the body, so it should be avoided whenever possible. It's so easy to flavour foods without this item, and there are lots of foods out there now stating they are MSG-free, as more and more people are becoming aware of this food substitute. The problem is that it's often not referred to MSG in the ingredients list, as it has about another 40 names it's known by. You can easily look this list up online to familiarise yourself with it, or you can simply avoid processed foods as much as possible. Then, by default, you won't be consuming it anyway.

Tap Water – Filtered Water

Most people's tap water is full of heavy metals, bacteria, and lots of not very nice chemicals. Consider investing in some sort of home filtration system to benefit your health and also make your water taste nicer (hopefully, meaning you will drink more of it). You will find a filtration system out there for every budget; they range from £10 for a table top plastic jar-type system, to thousands of pounds for an all-singing, all-dancing system that will produce water to every pH level you will ever need and more. As I am not keen on the idea of filtering water through plastic, and I know many people don't have the spare cash for the more expensive options, I have a recommendation for one that fits somewhere in between. My recommendation is the Berkefeld system (or a similar brand). This system can be picked up for a little under £100, and if you purchase their all-singing, all-dancing filters for it (which takes the price to a little over £100 instead), then this system will filter heavy metals, bacteria, and all the chemicals you can probably think of. It's amazing value for what it does, and it's set in a large metal table top system. That means no filtering through plastic; no need to constantly refill it, as it holds about 8 litres; and the filters can last for many years rather than weeks, like many smaller and cheaper options.

Caffeine-based Drinks – Rooibos Green Tea

There are some health benefits to drinking caffeine, but again that's when it's consumed in moderation. Most people have a caffeine addiction – if you are addicted then it's unlikely you are consuming it in moderation. Caffeine spikes the blood sugar levels within the body, thus upsetting many systems of the body (as mentioned previously). If you have hormone, mood, or energy issues, I would highly recommend you try substituting caffeine for another non-caffeinated drink, or by reducing your caffeine intake with green tea instead. Green tea generally has less caffeine in it than coffee and teas (but not always), and as it has far more goodness in it. If you have a bad time coming off the caffeine (i.e. caffeine withdrawal/detox symptoms) then you know you are definitely consuming too much, and it will in that case be messing with your normal bodily functions. Rooibos tea is a great caffeine-free tea, and there are tons of herbal and fruit teas out there now, as well as some healthy caffeine-free coffees like barley coffee.

Fizzy Drinks – Kombucha or Sparkling Water

Fizzy drinks often have sugars, sweeteners, colouring, and additives in them (among other things), so swapping fizzy drinks (even the ones that say they are sugar free, etc) is the best option. Kombucha is a great alternative as it's a fermented drink, so it's full of probiotics and other goodies. It can also be made to taste like champagne and even ginger beer (but without all the naughty ingredients). Another, perhaps easier, alternative to get hold of is sparkling water and then add in your own fresh or frozen fruit. I have had many clients break their fizzy and even caffeinated drink addiction by swapping them for this alternative. It's refreshing, healing, and tastes too good to be healthy!

Store-bought Juices, Smoothies & Concentrates – Homemade Juice direct from the Fruit

Unfortunately, many juices, smoothies, and concentrates are full of additional sugars, sweeteners, and preservatives. A great rule of thumb with this sort of thing is that if you can't see anything added within the ingredients list, then see what the best before date is. If it has a long shelf life, then it's more than likely got some-thing naughty in it to keep it from going off. Also, the longer an item is sat in the fridge/on the shelf, the less nutrients it will have in it. Fresh is best with this sort of thing, otherwise you could find yourself drinking dead calories – which kind of defeats the point of these items! Lastly, you can also opt for hot or cold water with some ginger, lemon, even cucumber in. This will make it a more alkalising, tasty, and cleansing drink.

High Sugar Fruits – Berries and other Low Sugar Fruits

As we will be helping you balance your blood sugar levels and the parts of the body reliant on this, high sugar fruits should be avoided or minimised where possible, as a large consumption of these will spike your blood sugars. By high sugar fruits, I mean any dried fruit at all, plus bananas, mangoes, pineapples, and papaya. Berries, on the other hand, are not only low sugar but also packed full of antioxidants, as well as other goodies. However, even the low sugar fruits will be removed for three weeks of this program (more to come about this later).

Table Salt – Sea Salt or Himalayan Salt

Standard table salt is really not very good for you. However, we do need salt in our diet, especially if you are suffering from long-term stress or anxiety, as the adrenals will be drawing additional minerals from the body to help them with the continuous fight or flight response. As such, opt for a good quality salt like a sea salt or Himalayan one, as they are packed full of minerals which the body can easily utilise.

Meat, Fish & Dairy – Always buy organic if you can.

As per the margarine/butter section previously, most non-organic meats, fish, and dairy are pumped full of chemicals prior to and during the processing part of the production. For this reason, it's always best to purchase organic and, where possible, wild. This way, you aren't consuming these chemicals and, hopefully, the animals, etc, have had a better life prior to being killed – which apparently (I'm veggie, so don't quote me on this) makes for a better tasting end product.

Vegetarian Meat Substitutes – Fermented options like Bean Curd or Tempeh.

It's surprising how many additional (and often unhealthy) things there are in vegetarian food, which unfortunately almost all meat substitutes are full of. Again, try to opt for items in a less processed state. Bean curd is a great option, as there's no added extras and it's fermented. So, unlike unprocessed soy, it's great for the hormones and much more easily utilised within the body.

Cooked – Raw food!

The more raw food you eat, the more essential enzymes you will consume. I recommend you aim for around 50% of your daily food intake being raw. This is actually a lot easier than it sounds. If you have a green smoothie for breakfast and/or lunch and a large salad with your dinner with a cooked protein option, then you are consuming more like 70 or 80% raw on those days. The more raw, the more enzymes and, also, the more nutrients you consume. It's really that simple!

Ready Meals – Batch Cooking & Freezing

Batch cooking is the way forward! Many people often fall off the healthy wagon due to wanting something quick to eat after a long day at work. My advice for this is to batch cook. Every time you cook a healthy meal, cook twice or three times more than you need that evening and freeze the rest down into single portions. Even if you only do this once a week, after a few weeks you'll have lots of different meals frozen down into easily reheated portions in your freezer. Just make sure you keep doing this once a week with a different meal each time, and you'll have an endless supply of quick and healthy meals to grab from the freezer at the end of a long day.

Microwave – Standard Oven or Dehydrator

Microwaves, although convenient, destroy much of the goodness within our food. Try and get into the habit of defrosting and reheating things on the hob – it doesn't take that much longer, turns out nicer, and preserves much more of the nutritional content of the food. And if you are willing to take it to the next step, then investing in a dehydrator (which dehydrates food so that it feels and looks cooked, but is still raw and has a much higher nutritional content and enzyme level) is a wonderful option. I totally love mine, and you can create some amazing meals in it with a bit of imagination and forward thinking (everything takes much longer to prepare this way).

Canned foods – Fresh, Glass or Carton

Canned foods (and especially if the can is dented or damaged in some way) leach chemicals into the food within them. If you cannot avoid canned foods completely, try to avoid buying acidic foods in cans, because the acidy of the food makes it more prone to the can leaching as it's more likely to break down the lining of the can. Almost all the foods you can buy in a can you can buy in either a glass jar, a carton, or fresh (and freeze for later).

Non-stick Cookware – Ceramic

Unfortunately, non-stick basically means your cookware is coated in a chemical substance, which will, over time, leach into the food you are cooking in it. Ceramic cookware doesn't have this added feature, lasts almost forever, and is easy to clean anyway. It may seem expensive to purchase such cookware to start with, but as purchasing ceramic means you will probably never need to purchase any new cookware ever again, it's actually a cheaper option.

Boiled – Steamed

Boiling food, especially to the point of mushiness, destroys most of its goodness. Invest in a cheap steamer, and steam those beautiful veggies instead. They taste better, look better, and are better for you; it's that simple!

Grains, Lentils, Beans, Seeds and Nuts – Soaked Grains, Lentils, Beans, Seeds and Nuts

Grains, lentils, beans, seeds, and nuts are all getting a hard time at the moment. People are concerned about enzyme inhibitors in nuts and seeds, and nutrient inhibitors in grains, lentils, and pulses. These inhibitors are what prevent the seeds, etc, of these foods from germinating in anything other than the moist ground. Generally, this is also the part of these food items that people react to and find hard to process, plus they inhibit our ability to absorb all the lovely goodness in these foods. There's a simple way around this, though, and that's to soak and/or sprout these foods before consuming them.

Once you have soaked them, you can always dry them out again (so they are crunchy) in a dehydrator, or at a very low temperature in the oven, and at this point you can also flavour them with herbs and spices. This makes a super yummy snack!

If you soak them until they have sprouted little tails, then you can use the sprouts in salads and other raw dishes, and you'll find you are absorbing much higher levels of nutrients in half as much food.

I have included a rough soaking/sprouting guide for you, below. As you will see, not everything will sprout, but those that will need their water changing every day to make sure they don't rot instead of sprout.

	SOAKING TIME	SPROUTING TIME
Almonds	10 to 12 hours	3 days (only if raw)
Adzuki Beans	10 to 12 hours	4 days
Amaranth	8 to 12 hours	1 day
Black Beans	8 hours	3 days
Brazil Nuts	3 hours	will not sprout
Buckwheat	6 hours	2 days
Cashews	2 to 4 hours	will not sprout
Chia	1 hour	will not sprout
Chickpeas	8 hours	2 days
Flaxseeds	1 to 2 hours	will not sprout
Hazelnuts	8 to 12 hours	will not sprout
Lentils	7 to 10 hours	2 days
Millet	5 to 7 hours	12 hours
Mung Beans	8 to 12 hours	4 days
Oat Groats	6 hours	2 days
Pecans	6 to 8 hours	will not sprout
Pistachios	8 to 10 hours	will not sprout
Pumpkin Seeds	8 to 12 hours	3 days
Radish Seeds	8 to 12 hours	3 days
Sesame Seeds	8 hours	2 days
Sunflower Seeds	8 to 12 hours	12-24 hours
Quinoa	8 to 12 hours	2 days
Walnuts	4 to 6 hours	will not sprout
Wild Rice	24 to 48 hours	3 days

The next things to consider swapping out are things within the home. When embarking on a standard detox, often little thought is given to what we bring into our home and also, for that matter, put onto our body. However, my wish for this program is to give you easy ways to reduce your toxic load moving forward, so that you do not find yourself in need of another detox at some point in the future. As such, swapping naughty for not-so-naughty with what we bring into the home has an impact on your own toxic load, as well as that of the planet. And if we can help the planet by helping ourselves, then that's even better!

Continuing the conscious purchasing for the home, as well as your meals, helps with this. As old and possibly toxic items run out, consider replacing them with healthier and less toxic versions. You'll find if you make many of the items yourself (which takes no time at all... honestly), it actually saves you quite a bit of money – winner!

Lots of different types of Toxic Cleaning Products – Vinegar, Essential Oils, and Sodium Bicarbonate (bi-carb)

Whatever comes into contact with your skin is more than likely being absorbed by your body, and if it's not being absorbed through the skin then it's likely being absorbed through your respiratory system. The rule of thumb here is: if you can smell it, then you are breathing it in. For this reason, even if you can't bear being without your normal cleaning products, try and opt for the ones that don't smell as strongly.

I have personally found that there isn't much in the home that some white vinegar, water, and a few essential oils cannot clean. It costs pennies, takes seconds to make up, and you can make it with your preferred scents. It only smells vinegary whilst wet, and as soon as it dries all you can smell are the essential oils. Pick essential oils that are naturally anti-bacterial ones for kitchens and bathrooms, and away you go.

If you have any stubborn stains, grease, or greyness in fabrics, then a little scrub with some bi-carb usually does the trick there. It couldn't be simpler!

Air, Carpet or Furniture Fresheners – Essential Oils and Bi-Carb

Simply put, air, carpet, and furniture fresheners do little to 'freshen' the air, and are incredibly toxic for our bodies and the environment. Use a selection of essential oils and water in a spray bottle, an oil burner, or simply sprinkle bi-carb onto carpets and furniture, leave to sit and then vacuum up. A little bi-carb in a bowl in the kitchen after cooking something smelly like fish, or in the car after you've taken your dogs for a wet winter walk, will eliminate almost all smells – it's amazingly effective, natural, and cheap to purchase.

Furniture – New for Old

Buy old, second-hand furniture, where possible. This sort of furniture was generally made with fewer toxic chemicals (unless lead-based paint was used) and the chemicals that were used will have, for the most part, already off-gassed. This means that the potentially toxic fumes created by its production will have already dissipated before you bring it into your home.

Single-Use/Flexible Plastics – Reusable or Non-Plastic Options

Where possible, try to avoid or minimise single-use plastics and soft flexible plastics, like shower curtains, tablecloths, and furniture covers in your home. These are full of toxic chemicals and, generally, the more flexible they are the more toxic chemicals there are in them. Also, they smell strongly when you first purchase them, which means you'll be breathing that in as well. Opt for more natural fabrics that you can wash rather than wipe clean, like cotton tablecloths or glass shower screens. If you can't do without that wipe-clean tablecloth, etc, then pop it out on your washing line in direct sunlight when you first purchase it, and the sunlight will help break down the chemicals creating the smell.

Rugs, Carpets, Curtains and Furnishings – Natural Fibres

Where possible, try to opt for items produced with natural fibres, etc. By this, I mean instead of nylon and other man-made fabrics, opt for cottons, wools, or even silks. They don't even have to be organic, but the more natural, the better, as the less chemicals they are likely to have in/on them. And the same goes for your clothing, where possible!

Washing Powder/Liquid – Natural Versions

Firstly, it's worth mentioning here that when we wash our clothes, we are all generally using too much washing powder/liquid. What happens is this builds up on our clothes and then, as it's next to our skin, it generally gets absorbed through our skin and into the body. So even if you can't bear to be without your normal washing powder/liquid, then consider every few washes not actually using any of said powder/liquid in the wash. This way, the residue that has built up on the clothing from previous washes will be used up and not added to. It will also save you money – another winner!

My favourite natural alternative to the standard and often toxic washing powders/liquids, is to use soap nuts instead. These can be purchased in bulk online, and cost a small fraction of the cost of standard powders/liquids. I buy a new bag every 18 months or so, and this costs me roughly £10. These soap nuts can also be composted, or saved up and used in natural shampoo recipes, etc.

There are, of course, lots of natural options in the stores these days as well, or it's super easy to make your own.

Poor Air Quality within or around your Home – Plants and Himalayan Salt Lamps

If you live near a busy road, factory, or you have a smoker or serial perfume/hair sprayer (ha) in your home, then there are ways you can naturally clean up the air quality within your home (or office). Plants are one of the best ways you can do this. They remove many nasty things from the air, and help purify it instead. Introduce as many leafy green plants as possible, especially things like Peace Lilies, Ivy, and Aloe Vera, and these will assist you to breathe in much cleaner and, thus, nourishing air.

The other way to clean the air you breathe is by purchasing Himalayan salt lamps and/or candle holders (or anything made from this salt at all). This amazing salt ionises the air, draws toxins from the environment it is in, and even draws dampness from its surroundings. These also look beautiful and, of course, are functional – another winner!

Scented Candles – Homemade, Natural Candles

It's generally believed that scented candles must be better for us than air-fresheners, etc. However, standard scented candles you purchase are packed full of artificial colourings and scents as well as petroleum, which, when burned, are released into the air you are breathing. Opt for natural, essential oil-scented versions, or

– even better – ones you make yourself from either beeswax or GMO-free soy. Candles are so easy to make, add in the scents you like, and they also make wonderful gifts for others.

If you would like to give making some of the above a go, then recipes for making your own cleaning products, candles, etc, can be found in my book *Living a Life Less Toxic* or on my website.

This week's nourishment chart is very similar to last week's, but now you'll be swapping the naughty for the not-so-naughty (as mentioned earlier in this chapter). This is especially important for the food items I mentioned. Out with anything that spikes the blood sugar levels, and in with the slow-releasing foods and drinks.

NOURISHMENT CHART - WEEK TWO								
		M	T	W	T	F	S	S
Morning	Meditate (or do this whenever it feels right)							
	Visualise							
	Body brush (after a bath or shower)							
	Green smoothie							
	Drink 2-3 ltrs of water (throughout the day)							
	Zinc							
	Magnesium							
	Zeolite Clay							
	B12							
Afternoon	Visualise							
	No caffeine							
	Make a nourishing lunch choice							
	Fermented veggies							
	No white carbs							
	No trans-fats							
Evening	Tapping (or do this whenever it feels right)							
	Visualise							
	Make a nourishing dinner choice							
	Fermented veggies							
	Add some seaweed to dinner (or lunch)							
	Epsom salt bath							
	No processed meals							
	No processed sugars							
	No alcohol							

Hurdles to Healing

1. If you struggle this week, remember that it's about swapping naughty for not-so-naughty, so any healthier choice is better.

2. Tap on whatever you are struggling with, whatever you are internalising. Get it all out, every single word, and then tap on being open to healing, letting go and cleansing.

Chapter 6: Week Three

Week Three is about maintaining and maximising detoxification whilst supporting the body during its detox, to ensure minimal detoxification symptoms. We'll be doing this by entering the yeast and parasite cleanse part of the program. During this part, it's important to follow the program as closely as you can to minimise the amount of time the yeast cleanse takes. The stricter you are with yourself during this section, the quicker you will finish the cleanse. Consuming naughty foods in this time basically means the longer this part of your cleanse will take you to finish, as with each naughty food you'll be feeding the yeasts and/or parasites again.

From here on in, this holistic detox program is all about inviting more balance and harmony into your body and mind, so the mind detox sessions (below) for this week concentrate on this concept. With more harmony comes more healing; when we fight ourselves and that which is around us, we only cause more conflict, and more conflict causes dis-ease for body and mind. This is an important concept to invite into your everyday life. When we feel stressed, anxious, or overwhelmed by life, we are not in a nurturing or nourishing state and, in fact, the only thing we help in this state is to raise our stress levels which affects our health and wellbeing. What if, just for today, you saw the stress, anxiety, and being over-whelmed, as an invitation to heal a little more of yourself? Use it to tap on, meditate on, or work through in some way, because I'm telling you nothing new here when I say we did not come to this planet to feel this way. Play with this concept and see how it can easily change your thinking about day-to-day events and make you less reactive to events, and, instead, use them as part of your healing practice.

Harmonious Healing through Tapping:

1. Start by saying the set-up phrase: 'Even though my body and mind don't always feel happy, healthy and harmonious, I deeply love and accept myself.' If you struggle to say this, then try opting for one of the other set-up phrases in the 'Getting Focused' chapter earlier in the book; or, better still, work on what's holding you back from saying this first.

2. Whilst saying this set-up phrase three times, tap the top of your head (see the 'Getting Focused' chapter for exact tapping points).

3. Now move on to tapping the other points in turn, as explained previously. Say out loud how stressed/anxious/ overwhelmed you feel, including where you feel them in the body, how they feel, even what colours they feel like. Use as much detail as possible. Get them all out whilst you tap, no matter how irrelevant; this will help you use them to heal and break down blockages and habits based on them. Keep going, moving on to each new tapping point until you feel everything is out.

4. Now it's time to start tapping on inviting health, happiness, and harmony in.

5. During this part, you may want to say things like this...

I invite health, happiness, and harmony into my life where there was once disease.

I am open to living in a more harmonious way.

I am open to letting go of stress, anxiety and feeling over-whelmed. I know it does not serve me, and hinders me, instead.

I may think I work my best under pressure, but I am open to working my best in harmony, instead.

I know I did not come to this planet to feel this way so I am open to the fullness of what I did come to this planet to experience.

I let go of all that does not serve me now, so I can live a more balanced life.

I let go of reacting to certain situations and people in a way that hinders my health.

I understand that when I perceive myself reacting nega-tively to something this is really an invitation to resolve something within, and I am open to doing this.

I listen now to the messages my body and mind are giving me to help me live in harmony.

I am open to living in health, happiness and harmony.

I get out of my own way and let go of the need to struggle through just because that's what I think is expected of me.

I am open to living in a more balanced and harmonious way.

I live in a more balanced and harmonious way.

I am more balanced and harmonious.

6. If you feel anything else come up, then please tap on this; just try to always finish on a positive and being open to healing note! Keep going until you feel you have got everything out. If you have been bad to yourself in any way, make sure to ask for health, happiness, and harmony in that particular area of your life, saying you are open to these things in that area of your life.

7. When you are completely done, take a few deep breaths, breathing out any residual dis-ease and breathing in health, happiness, and harmony.

Balancing with Visualisation

Start and/or finish all your meditations, quiet times, or even sleeps with a short visualisation where you fully embody balance and harmony. Violet is a wonderful balancing colour, so imagine your-self filled to the brim with light violet energy. You are the size, shape, and have the health you wish to have. You have all the will you ever need to achieve this. You are perfect.

Balancing Meditation

1. Find a comfortable and supportive position to sit in (pref-erably, don't lie down unless you cannot manage to sit up due to your health). Switch off phones and computers, or anything else that may distract you.

2. Breathe deeply and fully (making sure to expel all the stale air from your lungs and bring in as much clean refreshing air as possible) in through the nose and out through the mouth.

3. Now bring your awareness into the body as a whole (whilst continuing to breathe).

4. Imagine a beautifully balancing light violet light coming down from above and gently entering the top of your head where it heals the dis-ease and discomfort within the thinking brain, as well as the head itself.

5. Feel yourself letting go of the stresses, the anxiety, and overwhelm that does not serve you. Let it all go, breathe it all out. You no longer need this to function, to make sure things get done. They will or won't get done anyway. Everything is happening just as it should and when it should.

6. The light violet light is now making its way down into your neck and shoulders where you can noticeably feel yourself letting go of all that heaviness you have been carrying there (the pain and discomfort created within your body due to the stress, anxiety, and overwhelm you have been struggling with).

7. The balancing light violet light is now working its way down into your chest area, including your heart. Here it opens up your heart to living fully in health, happiness, and harmony. The violet light helps dissolve the walls you have created around your heart so you don't get hurt, so that you don't feel, and so that you don't let people in. It dissolves these now so that you can fully experience life, in all its glory.

8. You can feel your heart, your chest, and your presence within the world expanding. You are open to the love that is here for you and to giving it more freely to yourself.

9. The light violet light now moves down into your abdomen, where it cleanses all imbalances here and balances out all areas of your digestive system. Feel it working its way down, opening, strengthening, and balancing as it goes.

10. You can feel yourself letting go of anything that does not serve you here, anything that is blocking your health, happiness, and harmony, and that you may be holding onto.

11. The balancing light violet light connects you more fully to yourself, to your own sexuality and your own power, as it moves down into your groin area now. You can feel it opening you up and balancing out any doubts or insecurities, and filling you full of love for yourself.

12. As the light violet light works its way slowly down your legs, you can feel it lightening any heaviness there that's preventing you from moving forward in life.

13. As it moves into your feet, feel it connecting you with the ground, with Mother Earth, and the beautiful harmony of life. You are fully grounded in the health, happiness, and harmony of life, and you can feel her healing you as you connect with her.

14. Know now that you are fully held by life, and you only ever need to remind yourself of this connection to bring you back into harmony.

15. Be aware that your body is now full of the beautiful balancing light violet light, sit in this awareness for a while,

take comfort in the fact you have allowed this wonderful, healing, and nurturing time for yourself, and thank yourself for this. I like to say thank you three times out loud, but do whatever works for you.

16. Slowly wiggle your fingers and toes, and open your eyes. You may wish to take another deep breath now and let go of any residual stale energy.

17. Repeat this meditation technique at least once a day, but preferably twice.

The Body Detox Bit

As I mentioned at the beginning of this chapter, this part of the cleanse is about healing the digestive system. The main way we do this it to address any yeast/fungal/candida and parasite imbalances within the digestive system and, in many cases, within the rest of the body.

Studies have shown that around 70% of us have a fungal and/or a parasite issue in our digestive system, although I find that by the time clients come to see me it's more like 90%. Fungal issues develop over a period of time, and are caused by long-term stress, bad eating and drinking habits, drug use (both legal and illegal), antibiotics, steroids, oral contraceptive medication, or a combination of all of the above, in most cases.

Over a period of many years, some of the above bad yeasts start to take hold, which is often the stage when parasites join the party as well, as they love a good imbalanced digestive system to hang out in. Initially, you may not notice any symptoms/side effects of this, but eventually (sometimes years later) you may notice your health isn't quite right, that you have digestive issues, low energy and/or one or all of the below...

1. Flu/Sinus Problems/Coughs/Sore Throats

2. IBS/Upset Tummy/Constipation/Indigestion

3. Depression

4. PMS/Mood Swings/ Irritability

5. Headaches Migraines

6. Chronic Fatigue/Low Energy Levels

7. Inability to Lose Weight/Weight Gain (especially around the middle)

8. Itchy Skin

9. Poor Concentration/Feeling Generally Muddled

10. Skin Conditions/Acne/Eczema

11. Dizziness

12. Muscle Weakness/Pain

13. Food and Chemical Sensitivity

14. Low Libido

15. Thrush/Athlete's Foot

16. Poor Absorption of Nutrients

The reason for this is that as the yeast/fungus grows, it produces toxins which spread throughout the body. They can affect all areas of the body and especially the immune, digestive, lymphatic, and endocrine systems, potentially affecting your hormones and, for example, thyroid function and insulin production. The more the fungus grows, the more toxins it produces. Your body works hard to try to remove these toxins, but without some additional help, the body simply cannot deal with the fungus and its friends, the parasites, so your health may steadily deteriorate.

The good news is that what we are about to embark on over the three weeks will bring the yeast/fungus, parasite, and toxins level back into balance and allow the digestive system to return to health. From this point, you will not only notice many of the above problems subsiding, but you will also be absorbing nutrients from your diet better and, thus, finding that having a healthy, happy, and more harmonious digestive system has a direct impact on many other health concerns.

My recommendations for addressing this imbalance within the digestive system are as follows, and some of them you will have already been doing for the last couple of weeks – bonus!

There are many yeast/fungus cleansing diets around – some lasting years; some just a few days; some using pills and potions; and some not. The one I recommend is one I have used myself and have taken hundreds of clients through, and it lasts roughly three weeks (slightly less for moderate cases, and slightly more for more severe cases). I have introduced it at this part of the cleanse so that you have already started to make changes to body and mind, thus making the detox symptoms of the yeast/fungus cleanse less. If you go straight in and do this part of the cleanse by itself, you will often find that you have more severe detox symptoms as the body eliminates yeasts/fungus, parasites, toxins, and changes its food sources quite considerably.

You are still expected to have some detox symptoms during this holistic cleanse, but a lot less than normal, as you are not releasing lots of things all at once. In fact, when you do release too much at once, the body cannot eliminate it all at the same time, and often, it's simply moved around the body and then deposited somewhere else again. So, gently does it is the best policy for nurturing the body through a detox program.

The aim of this part of the program is to starve the yeast/fungus so that it returns to a healthy level within the body. The reason this only takes around three weeks, compared to many other programs, is because we are supporting the mind as well as the body to let go and heal. And also, because we are starving the yeast/fungus of all it grows on, as well as adding in some natural but strong anti-fungals. Anything you eat or drink within this time that feeds the yeast/fungus, will considerably lengthen the time you are doing the yeast cleanse.

From here on, this is what I recommend for addressing a yeast/fungus and parasite imbalance within the digestive system:

1. Remove all sugars. This includes fruit sugars, dried fruits, and fruits themselves, honey, maple syrup and agave nectar.

2. Remove all yeasts and fungus-based foods. This includes mushrooms, vinegars (including in stocks and sauces), blue cheeses, pickled goods, and alcohol.

3. On top of this, you need to cut out all items that create a sugary/yeasty effect in the body, so this includes all white carbohydrates, like white potatoes, white flour/pasta, and white rice.

4. Also, reduce your consumption of tomatoes and carrots in their cooked form, because they become sugary.

5. Whenever possible, when eating meat and dairy, purchase organic, because non-organic can contain a high number of antibiotics and added hormones that the yeast/fungus love. Any pesticides and preservatives on fruits and veggies are a little gold mine for the yeast/fungus also, so if you can't manage organic, make sure you wash these well.

6. If you feel you have a sensitivity to any foods, then these should be avoided during this part of the cleanse to help the body heal and let the immune system strengthen.

7. I know this may feel like your diet is becoming restricted, but where possible it is important to vary your diet, to assist the replenishment of essential enzymes within the digestive system, and to minimise issues with food sensitivities.

8. Drink at least 2-3 litres of water per day to flush out the yeast/fungus and its toxins, and to support a healthy digestive tract. You can make this water more alkaline by adding cucumber, ginger, or pH drops.

9. Drink as many bitter teas, like nettle and dandelion, as possible to support the liver to detox during this time.

10. If you can get hold of them, making a tea up of wormwood, black walnut, and clove is highly beneficial to assisting the body to cleanse from the yeast/fungus, as they are all anti-fungal and anti-parasite. If you are in any doubt, see a qualified herbalist who will advise you on how and when to take these herbs. PS – Sorry, they do taste disgusting, but they do the trick!

11. Add in as many natural anti-fungal foods as possible – these include oregano, ginger, garlic, and coconut oil.

12. Remember the body brushing from earlier in the book? Well, if you haven't been doing that regularly, now is the time to start, because it's going to assist the lymphatic system to eliminate everything effectively rather than your body just reabsorbing anything you shift during this time.

13. And if you haven't been having regular Epsom or Himalayan salt baths, now is the time to have some long soaks in nice warm baths with these wonderful salts, as they help draw out the toxins created by the yeast/fungus and detox itself.

14. Make sure you are consuming fermented foods like sauerkraut, kimchi, and Kavas at this point, as they are all highly probiotic and will assist in putting lots of good yeasts/bacteria back into the digestive system, as well as detoxing you from the bad stuff. Please avoid the fermented drinks like kombucha and kefir during this time, as these can often hold quite a lot of sugar unless you know what you are doing with them.

This Bit is Important!

I highly recommend the two following natural (yet very strong) anti-fungals. These items will greatly assist with the cleanse, and work for both yeast/fungus and parasites.

1. Grapefruit seed extract (not grapeseed extract) is highly recommended. Please read the label, consume only as advised, and start with the minimum dose. This isn't for everyone, so if you find this is too much for you, then please discontinue use.

2. Oregano oil extract is an excellent natural antifungal, but again it isn't for everyone, so if it's too much for you then please discontinue use. Please read the label and consume only as advised. This works better in liquid form rather than capsules.

Neither of the above should be taken long term, but they should be taken for a total of 12 weeks from this point. I know this is way beyond the end of this program, but this is because the life cycle of many parasites is 12 weeks, so this will help to eliminate these fully from your digestive system.

Some Additional Help

There are a few other things that are helpful during this time but are not in any way essential. If you feel you may have quite a big imbalance within the digestive system, you may want to consider some of these. But you should be able to bring the digestive system back into balance without them.

1. Zappers are wonderful little health aids. You wear it next to your skin (on the lowest setting to start with, and never above 12 volts) for 60 minutes in the morning, afternoon, and evening (a total of 3 hrs). Zappers draw toxins out, right through the skin – they kill many viruses, bacteria, fungus, and parasites in the body. They also help to ground you and reduce the effects of electromagnetic stress, because they are negatively charged. Zappers help alkalise and balance the body, and they remove everything from herpes to Lyme

disease. These are not recommended for anyone who has a pacemaker or is pregnant.

2. Enemas are very effective at removing yeast/fungus and parasites from the digestive system. Enemas are fairly easy to do at home, but in my opinion they don't get high enough up the digestive tract to completely remove all the fungus and parasites.

3. Colonics, however, do, and are a wonderful addition to your yeast-balancing protocol. I highly recommend going to a fully qualified colonic expert, preferably with a medical or nutritional background.

You will know when you have come to the end of your yeast cleanse as you generally feel under the weather during it, but on the day you are back to a happy balance again, you will wake up feeling much more refreshed (much like you do at the end of the cold). This is always around the three-week mark, if you have stuck strictly to the program. Some people get there in two weeks, if the imbalance isn't as severe, and for some it's closer to four weeks.

This week's nourishment chart adds in a few more things. The anti-fungals are very important at this stage, as is staying clear of any yeast/fungus feeding foods. Remember to also do the things that assist the body with elimination, like body brushing. It might be a good idea to photocopy this cart, so you can carry it around with you to remind you what to do when.

NOURISHMENT CHART – WEEK THREE

		M	T	W	T	F	S	S
Morning	Meditate (or do this whenever it feels right)							
	Visualise							
	Body Brushing (after a bath or shower)							
	Green smoothie							
	Drink 2-3 ltrs of water (throughout the day)							
	Anti-fungals							
	Zinc							
	Magnesium							
	Zeolite clay							
	B12							
Afternoon	Visualise							
	No caffeine							
	Make a nourishing lunch choice							
	Fermented veggies							
	No white carbs							
	No trans-fats							
	Anti-fungals							
	No white carbs today							
Evening	Tapping (or do this whenever it feels right)							
	Visualise							
	Make a nourishing dinner choice							
	Fermented veggies							
	Add some seaweed to dinner (or lunch)							
	Epsom salt bath							
	Anti-fungals							
	No processed meals today							
	No processed sugars today							
	No alcohol today							

Hurdles to Healing:

1. It is expected in this time that you may feel a bit under the weather from the detox. This is perfectly normal and won't last, but is a good sign that you are doing everything right. Everyone has different detox symptoms, so just because you don't have the same ones as someone else it doesn't mean it's not working.

2. Remind yourself when you are struggling to stick to the program that it's only for a few weeks, and will make such a difference to your digestive health and, thus, the rest of your health and wellbeing through your body and mind.

3. If you are struggling in any way, remember to tap on those struggles, those feelings, that lack of energy, those emotional releases (and it's likely there will be those), and/ or any other things going on for you. Use them to help you heal not just what's going on at the time but the self-limiting beliefs which may be behind them.

4. Be careful of stocks, sauces, and spreads, as they almost all have yeasts in them (either listed as yeast, or as vinegar instead).

5. Plan your meals in advance and remember, when in doubt, brown rice crackers or oatcakes with avocado, or some pate, etc, on is a great go-to, or even vegetable sticks.

6. Also, stir-fries with a protein and some steamed vegetables are also super simple, yet yummy, go-to meals.

7. Pick restaurants that cook their food fresh so you can ask for it without the sauce, etc.

Chapter 7: Weeks Four-Six

The next three weeks have been merged into one chapter for you, as they will all be the same. At some time over the next few weeks you will realise that you have finished the yeast/fungus cleanse side of things. For some people, this will be in as little as one week, and for others it will be at the end of the full cleanse program. Whenever you finish the yeast/fungus cleanse, please continue with the rest of the cleanse for the full six weeks as this is the optimum amount of time to fully heal the digestive system. Once you have finished the yeast cleanse, feel free to add fruits back into your diet so your meals might seem a little more varied and yummy!

As we will be continuing to support the body with detoxification, balancing, and strengthening during this time, this is what the mind detox sessions (below) will be helping with.

Sustained Support through Tapping:

1. Start by saying the set-up phrase: 'Even though I'm not quite where I want to be, I deeply love and accept myself.' If you struggle to say this, then try opting for one of the other set-up phrases in the 'Getting Focused' chapter earlier in the

book; or, better still, work on what's holding you back from saying this first.

2. Whilst saying this set-up phrase three times, tap the top of your head (see the 'Getting Focused' chapter for exact tapping points).

3. Now move on to tapping the other points in turn, as explained previously. Say out loud how you are feeling right now. This may be things like: I'm feeling run down; I hate this detox; my head hurts; I feel emotional; I want to lose more weight; my skin hasn't cleared up, etc. Whatever you are internalising in your head, even if it's unrelated to this cleanse program, say it out loud whilst tapping on it. Get it all out.

4. Now tap on the opposite of what you have just tapped on, which means things like this...

I allow myself to heal fully and completely.

I am letting go of all that does not serve me.

I allow my body and mind to become nourished and nurtured.

I no longer fight what is here to help me heal.

I thank my body for all it is doing for me right now.

I release any blockages and any old habits or negative ways of thinking, and open myself to being in flow instead.

I give myself permission to heal right now.

I surrender to the process and all it has to teach me.

I fully embody this experience and choose not to push any part of it away.

I may not have lost the weight I wanted to yet, but I am open to this happening as and when my body wants to let go of it.

My (insert health concern) may not have gone away yet, but I am open to this happening as and when my body wants to let go of it.

I am open to whatever lessons I need to learn to let go of (insert) that is bothering me.

Thank you, body and mind, for your protection, your guidance, support, and help. I now give you permission to let go of all that does not serve me, and become open to all that does.

I am open and accepting, and I surrender to this moment.

5. If you feel anything else come up, then please tap on this. Just try to always finish on a positive and open to healing note! Keep going until you feel you have got everything out. If you have been bad to yourself in any way, make sure to ask for health, happiness, and harmony in that particular area of your life, saying you are open to these things in that area of your life.

6. When you are completely done, take a few deep breaths, breathing out any residual dis-ease, and breathing in health, happiness, and harmony.

Nurturing Visualisation

Start and/or finish all your meditations, quiet times, or even sleeps, with a short visualisation where you imagine yourself floating in a bath of orange liquid. The orange liquid nurtures, nourishes, and cleanses you. It heals the digestive, immune, hormone, and respiratory systems, as well as energises and empowers you to move through this cleansing time and into full health, happiness, and harmony.

Nurturing Meditation

1. Find a comfortable and supportive position to sit in (preferably, don't lie down unless you cannot manage to sit up due to your health). Switch off phones and computers, or anything else that may distract you.

2. Breathe deeply and fully (making sure to expel all the stale air from your lungs and bring in as much clean refreshing air as possible) in through the nose and out through the mouth.

3. Now bring your awareness into the body as a whole (whilst continuing to breathe), and from your heart centre outwards, feel the flow of an orange and yellow rainbow of liquid, slowly pouring out and purifying, whilst nurturing your heart and chest area.

4. It pours like a slow, flowing river from this area into the rest of the body, going up and down the body at the same time, cleaning, cleansing, and healing as it goes.

5. All areas of the body are fully engulfed in the nourishment and purification of this orange and yellow rainbow of liquid.

6. Feel yourself letting go, becoming energised, healed, and cleansed, as it continues to flow.

7. It flows into the area surrounding your body, starting with the feet and moving up around you to form a rainbow of orange and yellow spiraling all around your body, until it gets to your head. This rainbow of orange and yellow purifies, heals, and releases anything within you that needs releasing.

8. Stay within the rainbow for as long as you like, or until you feel fully purified by its magnificence. Then slowly absorb the rainbow around you, back into your body and then back into your heart, but know it is always there waiting to help you whenever you wish to call on it again.

9. Bring your awareness into the full body, taking comfort in the fact you have allowed this wonderful, healing, and nurturing time for yourself, and thank yourself for this. I like to say thank you three times out loud, but do whatever works for you.

10. Slowly wiggle your fingers and toes, and open your eyes. You may wish to take another deep breath now and let go of any residual stale energy.

11. Repeat this meditation technique at least once a day, but preferably twice.

The Body Detox Bit...

During the next few weeks, it's important to continue to support the body and mind during the cleanse – and to form new healthy, happy, and harmonious habits to use into the future. One of the simplest and most effective ways to do this is to consider your breath and posture.

Breath and Posture

You've been breathing all your life and you're still alive, right? In fact, it's something your body does without you even having to think about it, so what's the problem? Obviously, we all breathe, but generally not in a very efficient way. We breathe far too shallowly and this hinders many functions in our body. The bottom halves of the lungs are around twice as effective as the top halves of the lungs. So, when we breathe shallowly, we are making the body work much harder to get what it requires. This can create respiratory problems, anxiety and panic attacks, tension, fatigue, weakness of our body's core, and hinders the elimination of toxins. Also, shallow breathing does not expel all the stale air properly: a little fresh air is mixed with old air which we've kept hold of. This gives our bodies just enough air to function, but not much more. We need to expel almost all the air with each breath for full bodily functioning, and for optimum detoxification. A classic example of this problem is when we are stressed, anxious, or overwhelmed. We tend to take short shallow breaths, but if we take long deep breaths our stress begins to subside. This relaxes our muscles, calms our emotions, and heightens mental clarity. It has a physical, as well as an emotional, healing effect on us.

So, taking time to think about and practise good breathing will not only help your body with detoxification, but will also assist health, happiness, and harmony within body and mind. Energy levels may increase, digestive issues could improve, your circulation will increase, and even concentration could improve.

There are lots of techniques for breathing better, and here are some of my favourites. But basically, whenever you think of it, take a few very deep breaths right into the belly. Start and finish meditations, tapping routines, and even visualisations like this, to promote better health.

1. Breathe into the stomach, the back, and the bottom part of the lungs, rather than just the top part of the lungs. Breathing into the back not only helps with physical issues, but it also allows you to address things you have tried unsuccessfully to put behind you.

2. Whenever you think of it, breathe into the whole body (not just your core), filling the whole body up with a deep cleansing breath, not just the lungs.

3. Belly breathing: When you breathe in, push your stomach out, and when you breathe out, let your stomach go in. I use this sort of breathing during meditations and yoga, etc.

4. Breathe out as far as you can, and hold it for a few seconds (your body is in its optimum state of transfer between carbon dioxide and oxygen here). Then breathe in as far as you can and hold this for a few seconds also. Repeat this a few times. This assists with the elimination of many toxins from the respiratory system.

Another effective way to enhance good breathing is good posture. This is possibly one of the most effective tools to breathing correctly and to supporting your body.

You probably remember at school being told to sit up straight, but you also probably have no idea why you were repeatedly told this. If you are slouched over or bunched up, this means the lungs, as well as other organs in the body, cannot work effectively. Just by sitting upright, you will notice that you immediately start to feel more energised and engaged. This is because the lungs can take in more oxygen, and then move this oxygen more easily around the body to perform its essential duties.

If you want more energy, want to lose weight, be able to concentrate better, have less tension within your body, and even help the digestive system heal, then practising good posture will more than likely assist this and many other health ailments to improve. It's so simple, yet so many of us don't consider it. Start giving these tips for better breathing and better posture a go, especially when you are not feeling tip-top, and see how much they help.

Toxic Skin, Hair, and Dental Care

I know we have already touched on the toxins in our skin and hair care, as well as cleaning products, but I just wanted to run over it again to help you minimise the amount of toxins you are continually adding back into your body in this way, and for you to know there are so many more natural alternatives out there now.

Research suggests that we absorb about 60% of what we put onto our body, and perhaps much more than this with dental products, and when your skin is hot and your pores are open, like after a shower/bath or when out in the sun. Unlike the food we eat, the products absorbed through our skin do not get filtered by our digestive system. Instead, they enter straight into our lymphatic system and are also stored in our fatty tissues, because the body does not recognise them or know what else to do with them.

Some of the many side effects of toxic overload are premature aging, poor skin and hair health, and reduced collagen levels. So, in fact, if we weren't using all these toxic products in the first place, we probably wouldn't feel the need to use more of them over the years to assist us to look younger. A nourishing low-toxin lifestyle will not only help you live in better health, happiness, and harmony, but will take years off you! Just so you know.

A good rule of thumb when reading ingredients labels: If you need a degree in chemistry to read them, then you probably don't want to be putting this product onto your body.

Our bodies have an amazing capacity to deal with and eliminate thousands of potentially dangerous items from their systems every day. However, when we keep adding more, their amazing abilities become impaired and we start to become overloaded and start exhibiting health conditions associated with this. Once you factor in the toxins in food, cosmetics, dental care, and cleaning products – and even in the air all around us – you'll soon realise that we are considerably adding to our toxin load every day. So, even if you can minimise this a little by making a few more natural and healthy choices, your body will be in a healthier, happier, and more harmonious state.

Decluttering

My clients are often surprised when I start talking about decluttering as part of their cleanse program, but to me it's a fundamental part of detoxing the mind (as well as the home – ha!). Decluttering our environment (home, office, shed, car, whatever it is) helps us to let go of things that no longer serve us. So much so that I have even seen people lose weight from just decluttering their environment, because they start to let go of what they have been carrying mentally, but then physically, too. When you declutter you make room for new amazing things in your home, but most importantly in your head. People who have been wanting new relationships, customers, financial freedom, careers, are all likely to find them when they start decluttering. We put too much of our own self-worth on what we own, have, and the attachments to things around us, rather than on who we are ourselves. Believe me when I say the practice of decluttering is so incredibly powerful!

I have listed some of my favourite decluttering tips below, but if you struggle with this concept then take your time, do a little every day, and tap on your struggle around this. It will help you to resolve whatever is behind the struggle.

1. Do a drawer a day.

2. Make a list of how you want to feel when you have completed your decluttering. Then write under each item a small task you could complete to help you get that feeling. When you are struggling, refer to the list.

3. Always start with the easiest and simplest area first. This will help you get motivated.

4. Have three boxes at the ready. One for the charity shop, one for the tip or recycling centre, and one for items to be returned to or given to others. If you have these always at the ready, then decluttering a drawer or cupboard a day is easy.

5. Give away an item a day for a year.

6. Ask yourself why you are keeping each item. *Is it useful, do you love it, or does it serve a purpose?* If not, why do you have it? Are you attached to it in some way that you could work on to help you heal?

7. If you haven't worn or used it in a year, why do you have it?

8. Do you need certain items to remind you of particular people or places, or is it all in beautiful memories in your mind?

9. Declutter as though you were moving to a new home soon. If you can't be bothered to pack it up and move it somewhere new, then why keep it now?

10. If you haven't got it repaired in the last year, will you ever?

11. Don't get caught up reading each thing as you declutter paperwork.

As weeks four to six are all the same, you have just one nourishment chart for this time. Please feel to photocopy it three times for these three weeks, or fill it out in pencil each week so you can reuse it the following week.

You'll notice that the nourishment chart is all about continuing to keep out the foods that the yeast/fungus and parasites like, and keep in the natural anti-fungals.

NOURISHMENT CHART – WEEK FOUR – SIX								
		M	T	W	T	F	S	S
Morning	Meditate (or do this whenever it feels right)							
	Visualise							
	Body Brushing (after a bath or shower)							
	Green smoothie							
	Drink 2-3 ltrs of water (throughout the day)							
	Anti-fungals							
	Zinc							
	Magnesium							
	Zeolite clay							
	B12							
Afternoon	Visualise							
	No caffeine							
	Make a nourishing lunch choice							
	Fermented veggies							
	No white carbs							
	No trans-fats							
	Anti-fungals							
	No white carbs today							
Evening	Tapping (or do this whenever it feels right)							
	Visualise							
	Make a nourishing dinner choice							
	Fermented veggies							
	Add some seaweed to dinner (or lunch)							
	Epsom salt bath							
	Anti-fungals							
	No processed meals today							
	No processed sugars today							
	No alcohol today							

Hurdles to Healing

1. If you are struggling to stay focused, tap on what's bothering you, how it's bothering you, and how it's holding you back, and then tap on being open to not being all these things.

2. If you are struggling for energy or focus, consider your posture and do some deep breathing exercises.

3. Remember that decluttering means making room for new things in your life and letting go of things that do not serve you any more.

Section Three:
Moving Forward

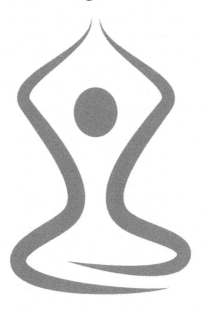

Chapter 8: Post Cleanse

Now that you have finished the cleanse program, it's important you don't fall fully off the wagon again and find yourself in need of another detox, diet, or program in the future. The tools you have learnt in the last six weeks can easily be assimilated into everyday life to continue to nourish and nurture yourself every day. Pick whatever resonates with you and whatever you have found easy to do, and continue these into the future.

For this reason, I have included another tapping, visualization, and meditation for you below. However, going forward it's important to do whatever feels right to you, so use these or a previous one I have shared, make your own up, or use someone else's – whatever feels right. But whatever you do, do something as it's easy to get out of the habit of daily mind detox sessions and they are so incredibly beneficial to mental and physical level. When we are harmonious in mind, we find it much easier to make nourishing choices for ourselves and we are much more harmonious in body.

Tapping for Moving Forward:

1. Start by saying the set-up phrase: 'Even though sometimes I allow life to get in the way of being nourishing and nurturing to myself, I deeply love and accept myself.' If you struggle to

say this, then try opting for one of the other set-up phrases in the 'Getting Focused' chapter earlier in the book; or, better still, work on what's holding you back from saying this first.

2. Whilst saying this set-up phrase three times, tap the top of your head (see the 'Getting Focused' chapter for exact tapping points).

3. Now move on to tapping the other points in turn as explained previously. Say out loud how you are feeling right now. Has the cleanse met all your expectations? If not, why not? Are you disappointed in yourself for struggling with it? Did you hate the process? If so, which bits? Have you found yourself emotional? If so, why? Are you worried that you might undo all the good work moving forward? Whatever you are internalising in your head, even if it's unrelated to this cleanse program, saying it out loud whilst tapping on it will help you to resolve these concerns of yours.

4. Now tap on the opposite of what you have just tapped on, which means things like this...

I am making nurturing and nourishing choices for myself now and into the future.

I understand I have to put my own health first, otherwise I cannot look after other people anyway.

I deserve all I am doing for myself, and more.

I love that I have taken this time out to do something for myself, and I will do more of this moving forward.

I am grateful for my body and mind, and I feel totally connected now.

I am grateful for the nourishing choices I am now making for myself.

I make more nourishing choices for myself each and every day.

I am grateful for my body and all it does for me.

I no longer put myself last – I am just as important as everyone else.

I invite health, happiness, and harmony into my life.

I give myself permission to look after myself, to listen to myself, and to learn from the messages my body is trying to tell me.

I will no longer ignore the messages of my body.

I will nurture my body and mind.

I am loving and kind towards myself.

I am loving kindness.

I am nourished and nurtured.

I deserve this.

I am health, happiness, and harmony.

I am perfect.

5. If you feel anything else come up, then please tap on this. Just try to always finish on a positive and open to healing note! Keep going until you feel you have got everything out. Be kind, be loving, and if you struggle with this then start

tapping on what you are struggling with and how it's making you feel, and use it as another invitation to heal something unresolved within you.

6. When you are completely done, take a few deep breaths, breathing out any residual dis-ease and breathing in health, happiness, and harmony.

Visualisation for Moving Forward

Start and/or finish all your meditations, quiet times, or even sleeps, with a short visualisation where you imagine yourself exactly how you want to be, in perfect health, happiness, and harmony. Make sure this image is very clear, colourful, and that you fully embody it. Imagine yourself looking the way you want to look, doing the things you want to do (climbing mountains, swimming oceans, or whatever this may be), and with the supportive people you wish to be surrounded by. Spend as much time as possible in this image, and as often as you can.

Connection with Mother Nature Meditation

1. Find a comfortable and supportive position to sit in (preferably, don't lie down unless you cannot manage to sit up due to your health). Switch off phones and computers, or anything else that may distract you.

2. Breathe deeply and fully (making sure to expel all the stale air from your lungs, and bring in as much clean refreshing air as possible) in through the nose and out through the mouth.

3. Now bring your awareness into the body as a whole (whilst continuing to breathe), and feel yourself centered and grounded in your seat.

4. Now imagine a light green light coming down from above, gently into the top of your head and slowly down your spine, lighting up, healing, nourishing, and nurturing your whole body as it moves its way down through every vertebra of your spine.

5. It then makes its way down your legs and into your feet, doing the same for you here, healing, nourishing, and nurturing you as it moves its way down towards your feet.

6. Your whole body is filled with this green healing, nourishing, and nurturing light now. Sit with this for a moment.

7. Now feel the green light moving through you and into the earth below, through your feet (even if you are several floors up, the green light connects you with the earth).

8. You are now connected with Mother Nature, and your green healing, nourishing, and nurturing light and her grounded, centered, and purifying energy are now mixing as one.

9. You can feel yourself fully grounded in this moment, fully embodying the dance between your body and her energy.

10. Allow her healing energy to enter your body through your feet and make its way up through your body, mingling with the light green light that fills your body.

11. Your body is now full of a light green healing, nourishing, and nurturing light and the energy of the earth.

12. You deserve this love, you deserve this connection and this support, not just now, but always. Fully embody this and you in all its beauty.

13. Now bring your awareness back to your grounded connection with the earth and know that this is with you always.

14. Bring your awareness into the full body, take comfort in the fact you have allowed this wonderful, healing, and nurturing time for yourself, and thank yourself for this. I like to say thank you three times out loud, but do whatever works for you.

15. Slowly wiggle your fingers and toes, and open your eyes. You may wish to take another deep breath now and let go of any residual stale energy.

16. Repeat this meditation technique at least once a day, but preferably twice.

The Body Detox Bit...

Going forward, continue to do the things you have found easy and/or the things you didn't mind either way about. By this I mean that if you didn't mind brown, quinoa, or sweet potatoes, then continue with these. If you liked some of the healthy meal options or found green smoothies nice and easy before work Mon-Fri, but can't be bothered with them at the weekend, then continue with the bits you found easy. Make some of the things you have done over the last six weeks part of your daily regime going forward, and enjoy continued and long term better health.

Being healthy can be as easy or as hard as you make it, but either way don't give yourself a hard time when things slip or when you aren't making as nourishing choices as you'd like. Giving ourselves a hard time only gets us right back into the fight or flight response within the body, which isn't a healthy, healing place to be. If things slip, then simply allow this, then ask yourself what is missing in your life at the moment, what you feel like you are gaining from the naughty food or habits, and use this as an invitation to resolve and move on from whatever this is. Tap your little heart out on this, and give yourself permission to just be you and to allow this slip-up to help you heal. We don't have slip-ups because we are weak or have no willpower; we have slip-ups because we feel that the naughty stuff is giving us something we are missing at that point in our life. This may be support, security, comfort, protection, company, or even love. See these slip-ups as good things that are informing you something is out of balance in your life, rather than your body and mind being against you; they are speaking to you and inviting you to heal this imbalance. Feel the body, don't fight it. Fighting causes dis-ease within the body. Listen, really listen to these messages from the body. Your body knows what's best for you and what you are missing, so listen, allow, and resolve, rather than fight. Then think of all that lovely energy that will be freed up from the fight to truly thrive!

And remember to be thankful for your body and all the millions of things it is doing for you every second of every day. This is especially important if you feel your body isn't doing what you want it to. When we focus on what's not going our way rather than what is, we block our body's ability to heal and to work effectively, because we create chemical reactions within our mind and body that create stress hormones. These hormones hinder our ability to heal.

When I began my healing journey whereby I cut out all toxic foods, cleaning products, cosmetics, people, I thought I had become well, but then soon afterwards I became toxic in my thought processes about my life. Everything had the potential to make me ill, I avoided so many things and constantly researched how bad living in the 'real' world could be for our health. Because of this toxic thought process about everything around me, I actually started to make myself unwell again. The world was against me! How could I be healthy when everything around me wasn't? What was I going to do?

I soon came to realise that the world wasn't against me. I was against me, and that was even more concerning and health-hindering than all the other things put together. When I worked on my toxic thoughts about being toxic, I let go of this feeling of overwhelm and my health returned fully to me. I'm not saying that we shouldn't take precautions about the toxic effects of a lot of chemicals out there, we soooo should. But what I am saying is that if you allow it to consume you, then the thoughts about this alone will hinder your health.

So, you can see now that sometimes being 'less toxic' can actually become toxic. Beware of your state of mind around your choices; if something feels off, if you feel conflicted, or feel like your body, environment, or the world is against you, then it's possible that there is something there to resolve. Tap on this, use this conflict, and know that neither the world nor your body is against you; you are deeply loved and held by both. If you do not feel this way, then use it to help you heal.

The mood/emotions behind everything we do have such a huge impact on how these things affect us. So, if you are reaching for a take-away or a beer for comfort, spend some time resolving this lack of comfort (through tapping or any similar techniques that works for you). Then if you still want the take-away, go for it. But at least you won't be consuming it from a place of lack any more, but rather from a place of treating your brilliant self to something yummy. When you eat a take-away, drink a beer, or consume anything 'naughty' from this place, it has a much less negative effect on your body. But when you consume it from that negative place of lack (or something similar), this will have a much more toxic effect on the body.

This fact is proven by the regular consumption of poison by some indigenous cultures around the world. Because they totally and fully believe it will not do them any harm, it does them no harm! (PS – Please don't try this at home, folks). My point is, though, that our mental state of mind has a huge impact on what's going on in the body, so nurture that mind and thus heal that body!

My top take-aways (no, not that kind) for maintaining a nourishing and nurturing life are...

1. Body-Brushing – I honestly believe everyone should be body-brushing daily, as it helps to eliminate those daily toxins you take on board as well as the added ones when you are naughty, and supports the lymphatics with the amazing work this system does.

2. Epsom Salt Bath – Well, why not keep something in which not only assists you to detox but is also a bit of TLC?

3. Keep as many of the foodie swaps in your diet as possible, especially any you don't mind. Why go back to something naughty when you can be nourishing instead?

4. Eat as much raw food as possible, even if you can only manage one smoothie a day. Every little helps.

5. Fermented Foods and Drinks – I can honestly say that even if you don't do much else, keeping these amazing foods and drinks in your diet will assist you to maintain a healthy digestive system, which then assists many other areas of the body. Have them daily, eat more if you are being naughty, and even put them on the side of take-aways (yes, those ones). They will help you to absorb the good stuff, digest the bad stuff, and keep the digestive system balanced.

6. Ask yourself when shopping and eating: is this nourishing or nurturing for mind, body, or spirit? Become a conscious shopper and eater!

7. Consider replacing some of your cleaning products with either shop-bought natural ones, or some vinegar, water, and essential oils. Not only does this benefit your own health, but it also benefits the planet.

8. Consider doing the same with your skin, hair, and dental products as well. With less toxins coming in, there is less you have to try to eliminate!

9. If you suffer with any sort of regular stress, anxiety, or feelings of being overwhelmed, consider staying off the stimulants and the things that spike the blood sugars. Your adrenals will thank you for this.

10. Listen to your body and when something feels like it is out, use that as an invitation to resolve something within you. If you ignore your body's messages, it will only shout louder next time!

11. Meditate, tap, visualize, or use any other mind detox methods which you have in your tool belt. Remember, they don't work if you don't use them regularly! Being in a bad state of mind is the first step to being in a bad state of body, and to making less nurturing and nourishing choices for yourself.

Feeling Blue List

My feeling blue list is one of the best things I ever did for myself, as it keeps me focused, especially when I'm not feeling in a good headspace. As someone who has struggled with my mental health for most of my life, I know how easy it is to slip back into a negative state of mind and to then make poor choices for my mental and physical health going forward.

It's surprising how when we are feeling low we can convince ourselves we are doing everything we could to make ourselves feel better. Yet in most cases, I'm sorry to say, we are not. I can't tell you the amount of times I've not understood why my mood has slipped, as I've felt I've been meditating, tapping, and doing whatever else is in my tool belt, only to realise later that my meditating was really me making a shopping list and my tapping wasn't on what I was internalising, but instead on what I thought would fix me.

One day after I had been feeling crappy again, I asked myself what I could do to break this habit. It suddenly dawned on me that something as simple as a feeling blue list was what I could do. So, I did it!

My list has evolved over the time I have been using it, and I have a version saved to my laptop and on my phone, so I always have easy access to it in times of need. And I'm telling you it really, really works!

What you do is to create a list (when in a good state of mind) of things you know help you when you are low (before the depression, despair, or darkness fully rolls in). The list should be in order of how much each thing helps you (the more it helps, the higher up it should be on the list), and it can include anything from meditating, to walking, or phoning a friend. The trick to the list is to second guess your low feeling self. By this I mean be aware of how you try to convince yourself you are already doing things when you are low. This is why next to 'are you meditating?' in my list, I have the question 'really?' because I know when I am low, I can convince myself that I am. The more honest you are about your pesky thinking brain, the more the list will help you.

Whenever you start to feel a little low, refer to your own feeling blue list and work your way down it until you are back on top form again. Allow your list to evolve as you do, and as you learn new techniques for better mental and physical health. And if you wish to add in things which you know help your physical as well as mental health, then you can call it your first aid kit or something similar instead. But whatever you do, just do it. You won't regret spending 10 minutes on this super simple mind-nourishing list, I promise you! I have many clients creating their own lists now and finding them incredibly helpful. Otherwise, when we are low, we can all too easily become consumed by the feeling.

I have shared my feeling blue list with you below so that you have an example that the things which work wonders for me.

What to do...	Notes
Are you Meditating?	Really?
	From a place of nourishment, or from a place of trying to fix, change, or improve?
	Perhaps you need to change your meditation?
	Have you convinced yourself this doesn't work, when you know it does, Faith?
You know you're enough, don't you, Faith?	If you don't, then use this as an invitation to resolve that feeling.
Are you listening to your body?	Really?
	Or are you just creating a list of ailments?
	Are you seeing the ailments as invitations to heal something unresolved?
Are you tapping?	On what you are already internalising, or on what you think is wrong?
	Go on, you know it works!
Are you willing to experience everything?	Or are you trying to fix, change, or improve?
	Conflict causes dis-ease you know, Faith!
Are you listening to upbeat music daily?	Or is it the same old songs on the radio?
	Are the songs slightly depressive?
Are you watching and reading inspiring/empowering stuff?	Have an inspiring movie day!
Have you taken yourself on a mini adventure recently?	Why not? You know you love them and they nurture you.

And here's a template of a feeling blue list for you. Print it out, fill it in, and save it wherever you feel would best benefit you when you are feeling a little low.

Feeling Blue?	
What to do...	**Notes**

I have included a nourishment chart for the post cleanse, just as a simple reminder of what you may wish to continue doing into the future. Again, you can photocopy it and use it each week going forward, or you can simply go with your gut and do what feels right for you.

NOURISHMENT CHART – POST CLEANSE								
		M	T	W	T	F	S	S
Morning	Meditate							
	Visualise							
	Body Brushing (after a bath or shower)							
	Green smoothie							
	Drink 2-3 ltrs of water (throughout the day)							
	Continue with anti-fungals for 12 weeks							
	Magnesium							
Afternoon	Visualise							
	Make a nourishing lunch choice							
	Fermented veggies							
	Minimal white carbs							
	Minimal trans-fats							
	Swap naughties for not so naughty							
Evening	Tapping on what you are internalising							
	Visualise							
	Make a nourishing dinner choice							
	Fermented veggies							
	Perhaps some seaweed?							
	Epsom salt bath							
	Meditate							
	Check your feeling blue list, if you need it							

Hurdles to Healing

1. When eating out, opt for places that cook fresh food so you can adapt the meal to your needs (almost everywhere that serves fresh food these days will do this for you).

2. When being naughty, have some fermented foods. They will help to balance out the bad!

3. Drink plenty of water to flush yourself through.

4. If you struggle, tap on it and allow the struggle to help you heal.

5. If you are unsure about something, feel stressed, feel overwhelmed, anxious, or even feel great – then meditate!

6. Use the nourishment chart, add your own things, and keep going with what you have found easy to do during the cleanse.

7. Make that feeling blue list if you are someone that struggles with your mood.

8. Instead of focusing on what you don't have, ask yourself what it is you want from life. I don't mean a new car, job, relationship, or home. I mean what you want on an emotional level. In my case, I wanted peace, but what I would do was focus on everything that didn't bring me peace and then create more chaos in my mind. But when I started to focus on doing more things each day to invite a little more peace into my life, peace came. So, what is it you really want for yourself? How much time are you spending on this each day? What can you do each day to invite

a little more of this into your life? This will not only help you achieve whatever it is you want, but less energy will be wasted on the perceived negative and you will also be empowering yourself rather than disempowering, which for many of us is our default setting.

Section Four: The Recipes

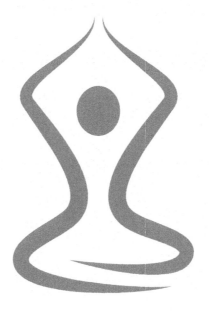

Chapter 9: Meal Options

The next few chapters are full of lots of healthy, hearty, and healing recipes. They are all wheat, gluten, yeast, dairy, and sugar free.

Pick the meals you like the sound of, write a shopping list, and make sure you have everything you require ahead of time. A good stocked larder makes for easier food preparation, and you are less likely to find yourself reaching for something naughty. With a little planning, the Cleanse Program will not only be easy but you'll find lots of meals that you may even like and want to continue using into the future.

Remember to batch cook when you find a recipe you like; make enough for several meals, and then freeze it down into individual portions for a nice easy and quick meal when you come home from a long day at work.

Enjoy!

BREAKFAST RECIPES

Brown Rice Pancakes

Make 2 pancakes

Ingredients

75g cooked brown rice

1 egg white

250ml unsweetened almond milk

1 tbsp. ground hemp powder

1 tbsp. ground flax/linseed

1 tsp. cinnamon

Coconut oil for frying

Directions

1. Put all the ingredients, apart from the oil, into a food processor and blend well.
2. Make mixture into two balls.
3. Add coconut oil to a frying pan and heat.
4. Add one of the balls to the pan and push down to make a pancake shape. Cook for a few minutes until lightly browned, flip, and then do the same on the other side.

Amaranth Breakfast Cereal

Serves 4

Ingredients

500ml water (or unsweetened almond milk)

180g amaranth seeds

1 tsp. cinnamon

1 tsp. chia seeds

Directions

1. Put amaranth seeds in a pan of boiling water, turn down heat after two minutes, and then allow to simmer for 20 minutes or until it gets thick.

2. Remove from heat and add cinnamon and chia seeds. Let sit for a few minutes to allow chia seeds to expand. Serve hot.

Baked Eggs in Avocado

Serves 2

Ingredients

1 avocado

2 small eggs

Paprika, to taste

Chilli flakes (optional, and to taste)

Himalayan salt or sea salt, to taste

Black pepper, to taste

Directions

1. Pre-heat oven to 350°F/180°C/gas mark 6.

2. Cut the avocado in half and remove the seed, then scoop out a little extra avocado to make enough room for your egg.

3. Rest the avocado halves into two separate, small oven-proof bowls, where they won't roll or move about.

4. Crack one egg into each half of the avocado.

5. Add salt, pepper, paprika, and perhaps the chilli flakes to taste.

6. Place the avocado dishes onto a baking tray and place in the oven.

7. Bake for roughly 15 minutes; this may be longer for large avocadoes and eggs, or less for small ones.

8. Optional: Add fresh herbs and sourdough bread to serve.

Breakfast Muffins

Makes 12 muffins

Ingredients

120g buckwheat groats, soaked

2 eggs

60g desiccated coconut

30g walnuts, chopped

30g pumpkin seeds

2 tbsp. chia seeds

30g flax/linseeds, ground

180g unsweetened almond milk

60g of any nut or seed butter

1 tsp. seeds from the inside of a vanilla pod

1 tsp. cinnamon

½ tsp. nutmeg

¼ tsp. Himalayan or sea salt

Coconut or olive oil for oiling muffin tin

Directions

1. Soak buckwheat groats for 8 hours in water and with a pinch of salt.

2. Drain and rinse groats, then allow to dry out again for a few hours.

3. Pre-heat oven to 350°F/180°C/gas mark 6.

4. Oil a muffin tin for 12 muffins, or several smaller ones that will make 12 muffins combined.

5. In a large bowl, mix the buckwheat, coconut, walnuts, pumpkin seeds, chia seeds, flax/linseeds, cinnamon, nutmeg, and salt.

6. In another bowl, add all the remaining ingredients and whisk until frothy.

7. Add the whisked ingredients into the large bowl with the other ingredients, and mix well.

8. Evenly place the muffin mix into the muffin tray – to make a total of 12 muffins.

9. Cook for 20 minutes and then cool on a wire rack.

10. You can garnish muffins with a little more cinnamon and/or seeds and nuts of your choice.

Oat and Ginger Granola

Ingredients

270g gluten-free oats

1 tbsp. chia seeds, soaked for at least one hour

2 tbsp. gluten-free flour

1 tsp. cinnamon

1 tbsp. shredded coconut

40g pecans, soaked for at least one hour then chopped

150g cashews, soaked for at least one hour then chopped

80g walnuts, soaked for at least one hour then chopped

¼ tsp. ground ginger

40g pumpkin seeds, soaked for at least one hour

¼ tsp Himalayan salt

1-2 tbsp. coconut oil

Directions

1. Preheat oven to 325°F/170°C /gas mark 3.

2. Put all the ingredients in a large bowl and mix well. Evenly spread the granola onto a baking sheet and bake, stirring occasionally, for about 30 minutes or until golden brown.

Broccoli Hash

Serves 4

Ingredients

400g sweet potatoes

175g broccoli (cut into small florets)

2 tbsp. olive oil

1 onion (finely chopped)

1 large red pepper (diced)

½ tsp. dried chilli flakes

4 large eggs

Salt and pepper to taste

Directions

1. Place sweet potatoes in a pan of boiling water, with a pinch of salt just for taste. Drain, once cooked.

2. Slightly steam the broccoli for 3 minutes.

3. In a large frying pan, heat oil over high heat. Add the onion and red pepper, and fry for 2 minutes or until soft.

4. Add potatoes to frying pan, and stir occasionally for 6-8 minutes until soft.

5. Add the broccoli and chilli flakes to the frying pan and turn down heat. Fry until the mixture is lightly browned.

Note: This goes well with poached eggs, scramble tofu, fish or meat.

Sweet Potato and Courgette Hash Browns

Serves 4

Ingredients

1 medium sweet potato, grated

2 courgettes, grated

½ tsp. Himalayan salt

1 small onion finely sliced

1 tsp. coconut oil

Freshly ground black pepper to taste

Directions

1. Mix the grated courgettes with the Himalayan salt and place in a colander. Place a dish underneath the colander and set aside for 10 minutes. The salt will draw the liquid from the courgettes. Squeeze the excess liquid from the courgettes until very dry, blot with a towel and place them in the mixing bowl with the grated sweet potato and onion. Mix well.

2. Taste and add more salt and freshly ground black pepper, if desired, then make into balls.

3. Preheat a frying pan over medium heat and add the oil. Once the oil is hot, add the hash browns. Press them down into the pan using the back of a spatula. Cook for 3-6 minutes.

4. When the hash browns are slightly golden, flip them over and cook for another 3-6 minutes.

5. Remove from heat and serve immediately, or allow to cool down and freeze for next time. I like to make up big batches of these so I have them in the freezer when needed. I then reheat them in the oven.

Note: Serve these with grilled tomatoes, tofu or egg scramble and you have yourself a healthy version of a fried breakfast.

Avocado Omelet

Serves 1

Ingredients

3 eggs

1 avocado, deseeded, halved, and sliced

1 small onion, chopped

1 garlic clove, chopped

6 black olives, halved (not in vinegar)

1 tbsp. olive oil

3 tbsp. fresh parsley, chopped

Black pepper, to taste

Directions

1. Add the eggs to a large bowl and whisk.
2. Add half the parsley to the eggs.
3. Add oil to a frying pan, and cook onion and garlic until softened.
4. Add the egg mixture and olives to the pan with the onion and garlic mix in it.
5. Cook for 4 minutes, and either turn the omelet over or pop under the grill to lightly cook the top.
6. Transfer the omelet to a plate and add sliced avocado to the top of half of it, then fold over and sprinkle with the remaining parsley and pepper.

Porridge

Serves 4

Ingredients

225g millet flakes or gluten-free oats

450ml unsweetened almond milk

Salt (a pinch of ground Himalayan salt or sea salt)

A pinch nutmeg or cinnamon

Directions

1. Put millet/oats, milk, and salt in a large saucepan. Bring to boil, then turn down heat. Stirring constantly, simmer for 5 minutes until creamy.

2. Place in a bowl and sprinkle with nutmeg or cinnamon.

See the smoothie recipes later in this book for more breakfast ideas. And remember, you don't have to have traditional breakfast things for breakfast. Salads, rice crackers, oat crackers, or poached eggs with some additional protein or sourdough bread are all other yummy breakfast options.

LUNCH RECIPES

Red Lentil Soup

Serves 8

Ingredients

300g dried red lentils

1 medium onion, minced

1-inch of fresh ginger, peeled and minced

3 garlic cloves, minced

1 tsp. ground cinnamon

1 tsp. ground turmeric

1 tsp. ground cumin

3 tbsp. olive oil

600ml of yeast-free stock

2 tsp. Himalayan or sea salt

600ml filtered water

Directions

1. Place oil in a large saucepan and gently heat.
2. Add oil and cook the onion until softened, but not browned.
3. Add the ginger, garlic, and spices, and cook for 1 minute.
4. Then add the stock, water, and lentils, and bring to the boil.
5. Reduce to a simmer and cook for 20-25 minutes.
6. No need to blend, but you could if you want it a little smoother.
7. Serve with sourdough or coconut bread (both recipes later in this book).

Curried Carrot and sweet potato soup

Serves 4-6

Ingredients

650g carrots, grated

1 pound sweet potatoes, peeled and grated

1 tbsp. ginger, minced

1 onion, chopped

1 lemongrass stalk, cut into 2cm pieces

1.5L yeast-free vegetable stock

500 ml unsweetened coconut milk

1 tbsp. olive oil

2 tsp. curry powder

4 kaffir lime leaves

1 tbs. Himalayan or sea salt

Directions

1. Heat oil in a large saucepan, and add onions and ginger and cook until soft.

2. Add carrots and sweet potatoes until these are soft as well.

3. Stir in the curry powder and cook for a further minute.

4. Add lime leaves, lemongrass, salt, and stock, and bring to the boil, then reduce to a simmer. Cover and cook for another 20 minutes.

5. Remove the lime leaves and add the coconut milk before continuing to cook for 2 more minutes.

6. Blend soup and serve.

Spicy Tomato Soup

Serves 4

Ingredients

1 large onion

2 garlic cloves

1 tbsp. olive oil

1 large carrot

1 large courgette

1 medium sweet potato

600ml passata sauce

1 litre yeast-free stock

1-2 tsp. paprika

1 tsp. dried oregano

2 tbsp. chopped fresh basil

1 tbsp. chopped fresh coriander

1 tbsp. chopped fresh parsley

salt and freshly ground black pepper

¼ - ½ tsp chilli powder (optional)

Directions

1. Finely dice onion, and then lightly steam in a pan with a little oil.

2. Crush the garlic cloves, take off skin, and add to onions.

3. Grate the carrot, courgette, and sweet potato, and add to the onions. Return to steaming the vegetables, stirring from time to time, until they begin to soften and brown.

4. Add the passata, stock, paprika, chilli powder, and oregano, to the mixture in saucepan. Boil and then simmer for an extra 15 minutes or until vegetables are tender.

5. Add the fresh herbs, and season to taste with salt and black pepper (optional). Simmer for 2 more minutes and serve.

Raw Cucumber Avocado Soup

Serves 2

Ingredients

1 avocado, seed removed, and peeled

1 cucumber, peeled

2 spring onions

150g cashews

150ml water

Himalayan or sea salt and pepper to taste

Directions

1. Leave the cashews to soak in cool water for at least 2 hours.

2. Drain the cashews and rinse well, then place in a food processor with the water and blend until smooth.

3. Roughly chop the cucumber, avocado, and spring onions, and add to the food processor along with the salt and pepper and blend until smooth.

4. Serve cold with fresh herbs on top.

Quinoa Falafel

Serves 4-5

Ingredients

250g cooked quinoa

2 eggs, lightly beaten

30g almond flour

3 tbsp. gram flour (or any other free-from flour)

1 large onion, finely chopped

4 tbsp. fresh parsley, chopped

1 clove garlic, finely chopped

½ tsp. ground cumin

½ tsp. ground coriander

1 tsp. Himalayan salt or sea salt

¼ tsp pepper

2 tbsp. olive oil

Directions

1. Add all ingredients to a large bowl, and mix well.

2. Make 24 balls out of the mixture, all roughly the same size.

3. Add the oil to a frying pan and heat. Add half the balls and fry until golden, stirring often.

4. Remove and drain on kitchen paper whilst cooking the other half, then drain in the same way.

5. Serve with a salad, fresh parsley, and a dip of your choice.

Quinoa and Edamame Salad

Serves 4

Ingredients

130g quinoa

1 red pepper, finely diced

200g shelled edamame

40g chopped walnuts, preferably toasted

1 tbsp. lemon zest

2 tbsp. lemon juice

2 tbsp. olive oil

500ml yeast-free vegetable stock

2 tbsp. chopped fresh tarragon, or 2 tsp. dried

½ tsp. Himalayan salt or sea salt

Directions

1. Toast quinoa in a dry pan over a medium heat, until it becomes to crackle. Do not allow it to burn. Rinse thoroughly with water.

2. Use the same pan to light toast the walnuts for no more than 4 minutes, and set aside.

3. Bring your stock to boil in a large saucepan and add the quinoa. Reduce to a simmer, cover, and cook for 8 minutes.

4. Add edamame, cover, and continue to cook until everything is tender, about 8 minutes more. Drain any remaining water.

5. Add all remaining ingredients, apart from the pepper and walnuts, to a bowl and whisk well.

6. Add the pepper and the quinoa mixture to the bowl and mix well.

7. Serve and top with walnuts.

Spinach, Pine Nut and Avocado Salad

Serves 4

Ingredients

60g small spinach leaves

16 cherry tomatoes

60g lamb's lettuce (or other soft lettuce or leaves of your choice)

30g pine nuts

1 tbsp. lime juice

1 tbsp. sesame seed oil

1 tsp. dried seaweed flakes

3 spring onions

1 large avocado

Directions

1. Put spinach leaves and lettuce in a bowl.
2. Cube the avocado, halve the cherry tomatoes, and slice the spring onion.
3. Toast the pine nuts in a medium oven or grill, and add to the bowl.
4. Add lime juice, sesame seed oil, and seaweed, and mix well. Allow to sit for at least one hour before serving.

Tortilla, Spanish-style

Serves 4

Ingredients

450g selection of peppers, onions, peas, sweet potatoes, courgettes, and greens

1tbsp. olive oil

4 eggs

200ml unsweetened almond milk

2 tbsp. rice flour

1 large tomato

salt and freshly ground black pepper

Directions

1. Cut vegetables into small cubes.
2. Put them in a saucepan with olive oil, and allow to slightly steam until they become soft and brown.
3. Combine eggs, milk, and rice flour, and beat into a batter, then season with salt and black pepper.
4. Put the vegetables in a greased flan dish or oven-proof bowl, and pour the egg mixture over the top.
5. Carefully slice the tomato and put the slices on the top of the tortilla.
6. In a preheated oven, 325°F/170°C /gas mark 3, bake for approximately 30 minutes or until the tortilla begins to brown in colour. Cut into wedges and serve with a salad garnish.

Raw Un-fried Rice

Serves 4-5

Ingredients

190g wild rice

½ head of green or red cabbage

1 red onion

1 tsp. cloves garlic granules, or 2 cloves garlic

3 tbsp. grated ginger (or half as much ground ginger)

2 heads of broccoli cut into small florets, stems peeled and shredded

2 large carrots, shredded

1 pepper (any colour)

1 bunch parsley, chopped, or 1 tbsp. of dried

190g peas and/or sweetcorn (frozen and thawed)

80ml olive oil, or your choice of oil

80ml sesame oil

½ tsp of dried flaked seaweed?

1 ½ tsp. Himalayan or sea salt

½ tsp. chilli pepper

Directions

1. Soak wild rice for 48 hours in water (changing water and rinsing rice every 6-8 hours).

2. If you cannot tolerate wild rice, or if you want a quick and non-raw substitute, then you could use brown rice, lentils or quinoa.

3. Put all vegetables (except broccoli, peas, and sweetcorn) and dressing items into a food processor, and blitz until all items are twice the size of peas.

4. Put mixture into a bowl, add the items you have left out, mix well and put into the fridge for 2 hours (or even better, over-night).

5. Mix well before serving.

6. If you don't have any of the above vegetables, use what you do have. This is a great 'use-up' recipe, so just about any vegetable works.

Roasted Vegetables

Serves 2

Ingredients

350g fresh vegetables, such as broccoli, cauliflower, radish, carrots, celery, and courgette

1 large chard leaf, sliced into ribbons

2 tbsp. crushed almonds

1 clove garlic, thinly sliced

½ red pepper flakes

½ tsp. ground turmeric powder

¼ tsp. ground cayenne powder

¼ tsp. ground curry powder

1 tsp. Himalayan salt or sea salt

1 tbsp. olive oil for drizzling

2 tbsp. sesame seed oil

Directions

1. Preheat your oven to 350°F/180°C/gas mark 6.
2. Place all the vegetables on a baking tray, drizzle with oil, and sprinkle with the salt, turmeric, cayenne, and curry powders.
3. Roast vegetables for 15 minutes, turning once halfway through.
4. Put the roasted vegetables and all other ingredients into a large bowl and mix well.
5. Serve as is, or with some quinoa.

Oriental Rice Salad

Serves 4

Ingredients

125g brown rice

2 tbsp. sesame oil

2 tbsp. lime juice

1 tsp. grated fresh ginger

30g flaked almonds (soaked for at least one hour and patted down)

30g sunflower seeds (soaked for at least one hour and patted down)

60g sesame seeds (soaked for at least one hour and patted down)

Freshly ground black pepper

Directions

1. Brown rice should be cooked until tender in lots of water. Remove excess water by draining.

2. Add lime juice, grated ginger, and sesame oil to the warm rice, and mix. Then allow rice to cool.

3. The almonds, sunflower seeds, and sesame seeds should be placed in a medium oven for around 20 minutes, stirring partway through.

4. Combine the nuts and seeds and lots of black pepper with the rice immediately before serving.

Vegan Fish Cakes

Makes 8 fish cakes

Ingredients

2 medium sweet potatoes, peeled

1 can of butter beans, rinsed and drained

1 large courgette, grated

130g gluten-free flour

25ml of sesame seed oil

3 tsp. of seaweed flakes

1 tsp. hot paprika

1 tsp. Himalayan salt or sea salt

½ tsp. pepper

Coconut oil for frying

Directions

1. Cut the potatoes into small chunks, place in a saucepan, and boil until tender.

2. Rinse with cold water and put in a food processor with the beans, sesame seed oil, seaweed, paprika, salt and pepper, and blend until smooth then set aside.

3. Squeeze out any excess water from the courgette.

4. Add the courgette and the potato mix to a large bowl, add half the gluten flour and mix well.

5. Put the remaining flour on a large plate, and heat the oil in a large, flat frying pan.

6. Split the mixture into eight equal pieces and roll each piece into a ball.

7. Roll each ball in the flour on the plate, covering fully, then flatten into patty shapes and fry for 3-4 minutes on each side until golden.

Vegetable Tofu Scramble

Serves 4

Ingredients

120ml and 1 tbsp. coconut oil, divided

1 to 2 cloves garlic, minced

1 tsp. sesame seed oil

¼ tsp. dried flaked seaweed

¼ tsp. sea salt

1 pack of firm tofu, drained

1 onion, chopped

¼ head of broccoli, chopped

1 pepper, deseeded and chopped

2 to 4 tbsp. torn fresh basil

½ tsp. fresh cracked pepper

¼ tsp. sea salt (optional)

¼ tsp. chilli flakes (optional)

Directions

1. Combine 120ml oil, garlic, sesame seed oil, seaweed, sea salt (and chilli flakes, if adding these) in a casserole dish.

2. Mix well, then crumble the drained tofu into the mixture and put aside to marinade.

3. Over medium heat, heat a large pan and add the tablespoon of coconut oil. Sauté onion and peppers until soft, then add the remaining vegetables and cook until lightly brown.

4. Drain the marinated tofu, add it the pan, and warm through.

5. Add in the basil and stir, then season with salt and pepper to taste. Heat thoroughly and serve immediately.

6. You can add brown rice or quinoa to this for a heartier meal.

Seaweed Noodle Salad

Serves 2

Ingredients

50g brown rice noodles

30g of dried seaweed of your choice

2 tomatoes

1 avocado

3 tbsp. sesame oil

A small handful of sesame seeds

Himalayan or sea salt

Directions

1. Soak the seaweed in a bowl of water for at least 15 minutes.

2. Cook the noodles, drain, rinse, and place in a large bowl.

3. Chop up the tomatoes and avocado and add to the noodles.

4. Add oil and seeds to the bowl and mix well.

Cauliflower Wraps

Makes 2 wraps

Ingredients

½ head cauliflower, cut into small pieces

2 eggs

1 garlic clove, minced

½ tsp. dried basil, or a small handful of chopped fresh basil

¼ tsp. Himalayan or sea salt

Directions

1. Preheat your oven to 350°F/180°C/gas mark 6.

2. Line a baking tray with greaseproof paper.

3. Blend the cauliflower in a food processor until it's crumbled down.

4. Place the cauliflower in a pan of boiling water with a lid on it, and boil for 10 minutes.

5. Drain the cauliflower then squeeze the excess water from it through a tea-towel.

6. Place the cauliflower and all the remaining ingredients in a large bowl and stir well.

7. Separate the ingredients into two halves, and make flat, round, wrap shapes out of each on the greaseproof paper.

8. Bake for 15-20 minutes (making sure they aren't hard, and can still bend like a wrap).

9. Allow to dry on a wire rack.

10. Fill with salad, hummus, and/or avocado, and/or a protein of your choice.

DINNER RECIPES

Polenta Pizza

Serves 4

Ingredients

For the polenta pizza crust:

110g polenta meal

1 tsp. dried basil

½ tsp. dried oregano

½ tsp. dried parsley

700ml of yeast-free stock

1 tsp. Himalayan or sea salt

2 tbsp. olive oil

For topping:

1 pepper, thinly sliced

1 onion, thinly sliced

2 large tomatoes, thinly sliced

1 bunch kale, finely chopped

3 tbsp. extra virgin olive oil

3 tbsp. sesame seed oil

For the walnut pesto:

2 garlic cloves, peeled

60g walnuts, toasted

2 large handfuls of fresh basil

1 large handful of fresh spinach

50ml olive oil, plus more if needed

Himalayan or sea salt and black pepper to taste

Directions

1. Preheat the oven to 350°F/180°C/gas mark 6 and grease two 11-inch flan tins.

2. Bring the stock to the boil in a large saucepan and immediately reduce to a simmer, and add the crust herbs, salt, pepper, oil, and polenta.

3. Make sure to whisk the ingredients continuously for at least 5 minutes and until smooth.

4. Pour half the mixture into one tin and half into the other one, and allow to cool on the side before placing in the refrigerator for 30 minutes.

5. Remove polenta from refrigerator and place on some grease-proof paper on two baking trays, and bake for 30 minutes.

6. Add all the pesto ingredients to a food processor and blend for 5 minutes, then spread evenly over the pizza bases.

7. Mix all topping ingredients really well in a large bowl, massaging all the oil and other ingredients well into the vegetables. Lay topping out equally on the two pizza bases.

8. Bake pizzas for a further 15 minutes and serve immediately.

9. You may wish to add your choice of protein to this pizza before baking the final time.

Pasta Ratatouille

Serves 4-5

Ingredients

1 small aubergine, chopped into small squares

1 courgette, chopped into small squares

1 sweet potato, chopped into small squares

2 small red onions, peeled and cut into wedges

2 to 4 garlic cloves, peeled and left whole

1-2 tbsp. olive oil

200g tomatoes (if fresh, chop into small pieces)

175g free-from brown rice pasta

Handful of fresh basil, chopped

Directions

1. Preheat the oven to 350°F/180°C/gas mark 6.

2. Place all the chopped vegetables and garlic in a roasting tin, drizzle oil over vegetables, and mix well.

3. Roast for 45 minutes, stirring halfway through

4. Cook the pasta, drain, and put back into pan.

5. Add the roasted vegetables, basil, and tomatoes to pan and cook through, stirring well.

Three Bean Chilli

Serves 4

Ingredients

60g aduki beans

60g red kidney beans

60g whole red lentils

1 large onion

1 sweet green pepper

1 large carrot

1 green chilli

1 clove garlic

2 tsp. coconut oil

600ml passata sauce

1 bay leaf

1 tsp. dried basil

1 tsp. dried oregano

¼ - ½ tsp. chilli powder

Salt and freshly ground black pepper

Directions

1. Prepare lentils and beans by soaking them in lots of water overnight. Before cooking, rinse and place them in pot with enough water to cover them. Boil and simmer until beans are tender.

2. Cut vegetables very finely. Remove seeds from chilli and dice, crush garlic cloves.

3. In a saucepan with coconut oil, place the vegetables, chilli and garlic, then slightly steam them or until they are soft.

4. Add the passata, herbs, spices, the beans and their cooking liquid, plus adequate water, if necessary, to make a runny sauce.

5. Boil and simmer until all the vegetables are tender and the sauce is thick. Simmer until the lentils and beans start to break: this will allow them to form a part of the sauce.

6. Season with salt and black pepper and serve.

Spicy Egg and Vegetable Fried Rice

Serves 2

Ingredients

150g cooked brown rice

1 yellow pepper

2 red onions (one roughly chopped, and one thinly sliced)

2 carrots, sliced into ribbons

4 spring onions, cut lengthwise

3 eggs

2 red chillies

3 garlic cloves

4 tbsp. sesame seed oil

Handful of parsley

Himalayan or sea salt to taste

Directions

1. Scramble the eggs in a wok or frying pan, and remove and set aside.
2. Place the roughly chopped onion, half the chilli, the garlic and sesame seed oil in a food processor and blend until smooth.
3. Add the above mixture to the wok/frying pan and heat through.
4. Add the thinly sliced onion, the rest of the chilli, yellow pepper, and carrot to the wok, and lightly stir-fry for a couple of minutes.
5. Now add the rice, stir well and cook for another couple of minutes.
6. Now add the eggs back in, the spring onion, parsley, and salt and pepper to taste.
7. Serve immediately.

Seaweed and Tofu Stir-Fry

Serves 2

Ingredients

2 strips of dried kombu kelp

1 carrot (and/or baby sweetcorn)

1 white onion

¼ tsp. chilli pepper

4 tbsp. sesame oil

Half a pack of firm tofu, drained and sliced into cubes

Directions

1. Add the kombu to some water, and soak for at least one hour.
2. Fry tofu in a pan with half the sesame seed oil, making sure to turn regularly until the tofu is browned on all sides. Set aside.
3. Cut kombu into strips, then do the same with the carrot and baby sweetcorn (if using these).
4. Slice the onion thinly.
5. Pour the remaining oil into a wok, and stir-fry all the other ingredients apart from the tofu and kombu. Add the remaining ingredients when everything else is cooked through.
6. Serve immediately, either on its own or with quinoa.

Lentil and Vegetable Curry (with optional egg)

Serves 4

Ingredients

200g split red lentils or puy lentils

1 litre water

780g selection of any of the following: leeks, onions, celery, carrots, courgettes, sweet peppers, baby sweetcorn, okra

2 garlic cloves

1-inch piece fresh ginger

1 tbsp. coconut oil

1 tsp. ground cumin

1 tsp. ground coriander

½ tsp. garam masala

½ tsp. turmeric

¼ tsp. cayenne pepper or chilli powder

¼ tsp. ground cardamom

Salt and freshly ground black pepper

4 eggs, not quite hard-boiled, shelled and sliced into four (optional)

Directions

1. Cook lentils for approximately 1 hour in water or until they are soft. Then puree them.

2. Grate ginger, crush garlic cloves, then cut the vegetables into same size chunks.

3. Put the vegetables in a saucepan with the oil, slightly steam for a few minutes, then add garlic and ginger. Steam longer until garlic and ginger are soft.

4. Add the spices and cook for another 2 minutes.

5. Add lentil puree and simmer for 15 minutes. Add water if it becomes a little dry. Add eggs at this stage and warm through.

6. Salt and black pepper can be added for taste. Serve with rice or quinoa.

Chickpea Curry

Serves 4

Ingredients

2 cans of chickpeas

1 can of chopped tomatoes

4 large handful of chopped spinach

1 onion, finely chopped

½ tsp. ground ginger powder

½ tsp. ground garlic powder

½ tsp. ground chilli powder

½ tsp. ground turmeric powder

½ tsp. ground garam masala powder

½ tsp. Himalayan or sea salt

Coconut or olive oil for frying

Directions

1. Rinse the chickpeas and set aside.
2. Add the oil to a fry pan, and fry the onion until golden.
3. Add garlic, ginger, chilli powder, salt, turmeric, and garam masala, and stir well.
4. Add the tomatoes and spinach, and stir again.
5. Add the chickpeas and simmer for 20 minutes.
6. Serve with brown rice or quinoa.

Black Bean Burgers

Makes 4 burgers

Ingredients

300g dried black beans, soaked, drained, and cooked

2 tsp. dried parsley

3 tbsp. finely chopped onions

1 carrot, grated

1 tsp. chia seeds, soaked in water for an hour

½ tsp. cumin

1 tsp. chilli powder

1 tsp. garlic, minced

40g gluten-free flour

2 tbsp. coconut oil

1 tsp. Himalayan salt

Directions

1. Put the beans in a food processor and blend, but not until smooth: mixture should be lumpy.

2. Add the other ingredients, except flour and coconut oil, and blend until smooth. Pour into a bowl.

3. Add flour, and form the mixture into burger-size patties. Place burgers onto a plate.

4. Heat coconut oil in a pan over medium heat. Cook burgers in pan for 4 minutes, turn and cook on the other side for a further 4 minutes. Watch them carefully, as they can burn easily.

5. Serve with salad.

Carrot, Parsnip and Cashew Nut Roast

Serves 4

Ingredients

450g carrots

175g parsnips

60g celery

1 large onion, diced

90g quinoa

125g cashew nuts (soaked for at least 2 hours)

1 tsp. dried thyme

1 tsp. dried sage

1 tbsp. fresh parsley, chopped

1 clove garlic, diced

1 tbsp. olive oil

Salt and freshly ground black pepper

Directions

1. Put carrots in a pan of boiling water and steam until soft, then transfer to a food processor and blend. Set aside.

2. Boil the quinoa in adequate water, turn the heat off. Cover and leave to absorb the water for about half an hour, and then drain.

3. Place cashews in a medium oven for 30 minutes to dry out. Do not brown too much.

4. Place onions, garlic, and celery in a saucepan with the olive oil, and sweat for 3 minutes.

5. Grate the parsnips and add to the pan. Cook over a medium heat, stirring occasionally, until light brown.

6. Combine all the ingredients with the carrots, and mix well. Season with salt and black pepper.

7. Place in a greased loaf tin, cover with foil, and bake in a preheated oven at 180°C/350°F/gas mark 4 for approximately 40 minutes.

8. Serve with salad or vegetables.

Protein-packed Baked Sweet Potatoes

Serves 4

Ingredients

4 sweet potatoes

1 small onion, thinly sliced

1 garlic clove, minced

1 can of white beans, cooked, drained, and rinsed

1 large bunch of kale, sliced thinly

1 large handful of parsley

¼ tsp. red pepper flakes

2 tbsp. olive oil

Himalayan or seas salt and pepper to taste

Directions

1. Preheat the oven to 350°F/180°C/gas mark 6.

2. Prick the sweet potatoes with a fork and place them on a baking tray, and bake for about an hour.

3. About 15 minutes before the sweet potatoes will be ready, start to prepare the filling.

4. In a large saucepan, heat the oil and cook the onions until soft but not brown.

5. Add the garlic, parsley, and pepper flakes, and stir well.

6. Now add the beans and cook for a few minutes longer, then add the kale and salt and pepper and cook for a further 5-7 minutes, stirring occasionally.

7. Take the potatoes out of the oven, slice them open and add the bean mixture into them and serve immediately.

Vegetarian Haggis

Serves 4-5

Ingredients

1 white onion, finely chopped

2 cloves garlic, finely sliced

30ml olive oil

½ tin of red kidney beans, well cooked and rinsed

Pinch of cayenne pepper or chilli powder

½ tsp. ground cinnamon

½ tsp. allspice, ground

Pinch of nutmeg

3 carrots, grated

75g red lentils

500ml yeast-free vegetable stock

Small bunch rosemary, strip the leaves and chop them finely

Small bunch thyme, leaves stripped

50g gluten-free oatmeal or oat bran

Directions

1. In a medium-sized casserole, sweat the onions and garlic in the oil until soft.

2. Add the mushrooms (if using) and sauté until light brown.

3. Add the spices and continue cooking for a few minutes. Then add carrots, lentils, and pour the stock into the pan, just covering the ingredients. Simmer, covered, until the lentils are soft.

4. Mash the beans roughly with a fork, then add them and the oatmeal to the pan. Add a little more stock if you think it's needed. The oatmeal should absorb the last of the stock: if it doesn't, then cook for a little longer. Season to taste.

5. Spoon out the haggis and serve with tatties (potatoes – sweet potatoes work just as well as white potatoes here) and neeps (turnips), and/or gluten-free oatcakes.

Living (Raw) Lasagna

Serves 6

Ingredients

1 large courgette

1 small aubergine

Cashew cheese:

200g cashews

1/4 tsp of dried garlic

2 tbsp. of sesame seed oil

1/4 tsp of seaweed flakes

1 tbsp. dried rosemary

1 pinch Himalayan or sea salt

50-100ml of water

Pesto:

1/2 head of broccoli

4-6 tomatoes

8-10 sun dried tomatoes (in oil)

1 large bunch of basil

A pinch Himalayan or sea salt

50-100ml of water

Directions

6. Slice the courgettes and aubergine very thinly on a mandolin or with a knife, and place in a little salt water for 30 minutes, then allow to dry out fully on some kitchen paper.

7. Make the cheese: Place all cheese ingredients in the food processor, blend until smooth, and add water until it resembles a thick sauce. Pour into a separate jug.

8. Make the pesto: Place all pesto ingredients in the food processor, blend until smooth and thick, add water until it's a thick sauce.

9. Layer courgette, pesto, cheese, and aubergine, in a small baking or casserole dish.

10. Leave to marinade in the fridge for 2-4 hours.

11. Optional: Place in a dehydrator for 2-4 hours if you wish to serve the lasagna warm.

SNACK RECIPES

Cauliflower Crackers

Makes 36

Ingredients

30g cauliflower, roughly chopped

50ml sesame seeds

70g flax/linseeds ground

2 tbsp. chia seeds

100g sesame seeds for topping

1 tsp. Himalayan or sea salt

75ml cup water

3 tbsp. coconut oil, melted

Directions

1. Blend the cauliflower in a food processor until it is well crumbled.
2. Now add all the other ingredients, and pulse for a bit longer until it forms a dough. Chill for 4 hours.
3. Preheat the oven to 350°F/180°C/gas mark 6, and place some greaseproof paper on a baking tray.
4. Make 36 small balls from the dough, and roll the balls in the sesame seeds.
5. Place the balls on the greaseproof paper and flatten out to make cracker shapes.
6. Bake for 30 minutes and then turn crackers over and bake for another 30 minutes.
7. Allow to cool on a wire rack.
8. Serve with pate, hummus, or avocado.

Spiced Potato Wedges with Garlic Mayonnaise Dip

Serves 4

Ingredients

4 medium baking potatoes

2 tbsp. olive oil

¼ tsp. chilli powder

Salt and freshly ground black pepper

Chopped fresh herbs, to garnish

Garlic Mayonnaise (see Side Dishes recipes)

Directions

1. Cut the potatoes in half lengthways, and then cut each half into four wedges lengthways.

2. In a large bowl, mix together olive oil and chilli powder, and season with salt and pepper.

3. Toss the potato wedges in the oil mixture until well coated.

4. Put the potatoes on a large baking tray and bake in a preheated 200°C/400°F/gas mark 6 oven for approximately 40 minutes, or until brown and crisp on the outside, but soft on the inside.

5. Serve with fresh herbs and garlic mayo dip.

Nori Vegetable Rolls

Makes 8 rolls

Ingredients

300g sunflower seeds (soaked at least 4 hours)

1 tbsp. dried seaweed

Half a bunch of spring onions

3 tsp. minced garlic

2 spring onions, chopped

180g spinach, chopped

8 sheets raw nori (untoasted)

2 carrots, thinly sliced lengthways

1 large cucumber or courgette, thinly sliced lengthways

1 large avocado, thinly sliced lengthways

Directions

1. Put first five ingredients into a food processor, and process until smooth.

2. Place on each nori sheet a layer of spinach leaves, sunflower mix, and then slices of carrot, cucumber, and avocado, along the edge closest to you.

3. Tightly roll the nori sheet into a sausage shape, and seal the edge with a little warm water.

4. Slice into small discs.

5. Serve with salad and dips.

Oven-Roasted Kale Chips

Serves 4

Ingredients

1 large bunch of kale

40g coconut oil, melted

2 tbsp. sesame seed oil

½ tsp. garlic powder

½ tsp. red chilli flakes

1 tsp. Himalayan or sea salt

Black pepper, ground to taste

Directions

1. Preheat oven to 350°F/180°C/gas mark 6.

2. Rinse kale, and dry out completely.

3. Remove any woody stems, and place the rest of the kale in a large bowl.

4. Place the rest of the ingredients in the bowl, and massage well into the kale.

5. Put the kale mixture on a baking tray and cook for 5 minutes, then stir well and return to oven for a further 5 minutes.

6. Serve as a snack or on the side of a salad.

Pumpkin Seed Oat Biscuits

Makes 18 biscuits

Ingredients

90g oat bran

30g pumpkin seeds

20g pumpkin seeds, to be added separately

45g almond flour

55g coconut oil, melted

45g arrowroot powder

55g unsweetened almond milk

⅛ tsp. cayenne powder

½ tsp. dried thyme leaves

¼ tsp. Himalayan or sea salt

Directions

1. Preheat oven to 350°F/180°C/gas mark 6, and place some greaseproof paper on a baking tray.
2. Add the oat bran and the 30gs of pumpkin seeds to a food processor, and blend for no more than 30 seconds.
3. Now add the almond flour, arrowroot, salt, cayenne, and thyme, and just blend long enough so everything is well mixed.
4. Place all the blended ingredients in a large bowl, and add the coconut oil. Rub mixture between your figures to make bread-crumbs.
5. Add the almond milk, and mix together to form a dough.
6. Add the remaining pumpkin seeds.
7. Roll dough out between two pieces of greaseproof paper until roughly ¼ -inch thick, and cut into biscuit shapes of your choosing.

8. Bake for 15 minutes. The biscuit edges should be golden, but not browned.

9. Allow to cool on a wire rack.

Coconut & Chocolate Macaroons

Makes 10 macaroons

Ingredients

300g desiccated coconut

60g warm water

60g coconut oil, melted

3 eggs, beaten

60g raw cacao powder, optional

2-3 tbsp. alcohol-free vanilla extract

Directions

1. Preheat oven to 350°F/180°C/gas mark 6, and place some greaseproof paper on a baking tray.

2. Place the coconut, warm water, and melted oil into a bowl, and stir well.

3. Whisk the eggs in a separate bowl, then add to the coconut mixture and stir in well.

4. Add the vanilla and cacao powder to the mixture and stir well.

5. Place a dessertspoonful of mix onto the greaseproof paper at 3 inch intervals, and bake for 15 minutes.

6. Allow to cool on a wire rack.

Sweet Potato Cookies

Ingredients

380g gluten-free oat flour

½ tsp. cardamom

2 tsp. ground cinnamon

1 tsp. ground nutmeg

1 large sweet potato, roasted, peeled, and mashed

120ml coconut oil, melted

180ml unsweetened coconut milk

2 tsp. alcohol-free vanilla extract

1 tsp. baking soda

¾ tsp. Himalayan salt

Directions

1. Preheat oven to 350°F/180°C/gas mark 4.

2. Oil a cookie sheet with a little coconut oil.

3. Mix together the dry ingredients in a bowl. Add wet ingredients and mix well by hand, or on the slow speed of a food processor.

4. Make 10-12 cookie shapes out of the batter, and place on cookie sheets in the middle of the oven.

5. Bake for about 20-22 minutes until cookies are golden brown and crumbly. Transfer to a wire rack to cool.

Chocolate Bites

Makes roughly 32 bites

Ingredients

325g coconut oil, melted

220g of any nut or seed butter

140g cacao powder

2 tbsp. alcohol-free vanilla extract

Directions

1. In a bowl, stir the coconut oil, nut butter, cacao powder, and vanilla together until well mixed.
2. Pour into ice cube trays or small moulds, and freeze for at least one hour.
3. Store in freezer and pop out of the tray 10/15 minutes before needed.

SIDE DISHES RECIPES

Coconut Bread

Makes 1 loaf

Ingredients

65g buckwheat flour

65g coconut flour

5 eggs

150ml coconut milk

2 tbsp. coconut oil

½ tsp. Himalayan or sea salt

1 tsp. baking powder

Directions

1. Preheat oven to 350°F/180°C/gas mark 4 and grease a bread tin with the coconut oil.

2. Mix the eggs, coconut oil, and salt in a large bowl.

3. Now add the buckwheat flour, coconut flour, coconut milk, and baking powder to the bowl and whisk until smooth.

4. Pour into the bread tin and bake for 30 minutes, until golden on top.

5. Allow to cool on a wire rack.

Eggless- Egg Salad

Serves 2-3

Ingredients

3 celery stalks, finely chopped

1 red pepper, finely chopped

½ small white onion, finely chopped (optional)

350g cashews

175 ml water

15 ml lemon juice

1 tbsp. turmeric

1 clove garlic

1 tsp. Himalayan or sea salt

Paprika, to garnish/taste

Directions

1. Put all ingredients, except the celery and the pepper, into a food processor and blend until smooth.

2. Put the celery, pepper, and onion (if you are using one) into a large bowl, and pour in the cashew mixture from your food processor and mix well.

3. Serve with salad, wraps, or on crackers with a sprinkling of paprika.

Marinated Vegetables

Serves 4

Ingredients

1 large courgette

1 red pepper

1 yellow pepper

1 small red onion

½ a small aubergine

2 tbsp. olive oil

2 tbsp. sesame seed oil

½ tsp. garlic granules

½ tbsp. mixed dried herbs, or 50g fresh herbs chopped

1 tsp. flax seed oil (optional)

Directions

1. Slice all the vegetables very thinly and add to a large flat bowl.

2. Add all the other ingredients to the bowl and mix well.

3. Cover and place in the fridge to marinate for at least 2 hours, but preferably overnight.

4. Serve with a protein of your choice.

Aubergine and Sun-Dried Tomato Pâté/Dip

Serves 4

Ingredients

1 medium aubergine

1 heaped tbsp. light tahini

5-6 large sun-dried tomatoes, chopped

1 clove garlic, chopped

2 tsp. olive oil

1 tsp. fresh chives, chopped

1 tsp. fresh thyme, chopped

Salt and pepper to taste

Directions

1. Wrap the aubergine in foil paper and bake in a medium heat oven for 1 hour or until soft. Allow to cool, then cut into chunks.

2. Put aubergine, sun-dried tomatoes, garlic, olive oil, tahini, and fresh herbs into a food processor and blend until smooth.

3. Put mixture into a pan, heat through for 10 minutes and season to taste.

Guacamole

Ingredients

½ red onion, finely chopped

1 tsp. finely chopped garlic

50-100g coarsely chopped tomato

2 large avocadoes, peeled, pitted, and cut into chunks

1 tsp. fresh lime juice

¼ tsp. cumin (optional)

Salt and pepper to taste

Directions

1. Cut the onion, garlic, and tomato and place in a bowl. Crush the avocadoes, squeeze the lime over the top, and add the cumin.

2. Add salt and pepper.

White Bean Purée

Serves 2-4 as a side

Ingredients

1 black-eyed peas, cooked, drained, and rinsed well

2 garlic cloves, minced

2 tbsp. fresh parsley, chopped

1 tsp. cumin powder

1 tsp. chilli powder

2 tbsp. olive oil

150ml water, more if needed

2 tsp. Himalayan or sea salt

Directions

1. Place all ingredients into a food processor and blend until smooth.

2. Serve immediately or store in refrigerator.

Nut or Seed Butters

Ingredients

700g nuts or seeds, soaked (as per the soaking table earlier in this book) and dried

½ tsp. Himalayan or sea salt

2 tbsp. olive oil

Directions

1. Place nuts or seeds into a high-powered food processor.
2. Add salt and oil, and blend for 15 minutes.
3. Stop blending occasionally to push all the extra nut/seed mix down around the edges of the blender and to allow the machine to cool a little.
4. After 15 minutes, you'll end up with a nut butter to spread on crackers, breads, or even on potatoes.

Hummus and Grated Carrot Paste

Serves 4-6

Ingredients

225g carrots

225g cooked chickpeas

3 tbsp. light tahini

2 spring onions

1 tbsp. olive oil

Fresh herbs, to garnish

Directions

1. Grate carrots finely.
2. Put the remaining ingredients, except the fresh herbs, in a food processor and process until the mixture becomes silky smooth.
3. Add water if needed, to ensure you get the desired texture.
4. Add the carrots to the hummus, mix thoroughly, and garnish with fresh herbs. Serve with a small salad and/or gluten-free crackers.

Garlic Mayonnaise

Ingredients

1-2 cloves garlic, crushed

290g packet silken tofu

180ml filtered water

30-50ml olive oil

Salt and freshly ground black pepper

Directions

1. Add all the ingredients, except the oil, to a food processor and blend until smooth.
2. Add oil slowly until it is the right mayonnaise texture.
3. Season to taste, and place in a refrigerator for 1-2 hours before serving.

Gravy

Ingredients

1.5 tbsp. olive oil

½ -1 white onion, chopped

1 small clove garlic, minced or grated

1 tbsp. gluten-free flour

300-400ml yeast-free stock vegetable stock

Salt and pepper to taste

Directions

1. Add oil to a heated saucepan.
2. Add onion and cook through, add garlic and cook until lightly brown.
3. Stir in flour and then slowly add vegetable stock and stir until thickened (if you add the stock too quickly, you'll get lumps).

Chapter 10: Drink Options

Green Smoothies

Green Smoothie

Ingredients

1 avocado, peeled and deseeded

2 stalks of celery, chopped

½ large cucumber, chopped

3-4 basil leaves

¼ of a clove of garlic

¼ tsp Himalayan salt

A handful of parsley

Water

Directions

1. Place all the ingredients in a blender, and top up with water.
2. Blend until smooth.

Alternative Green Smoothie

Ingredients

500ml of unsweetened almond milk

1 avocado, peeled and deseeded

1 large handful of spinach

½ a small cucumber, chopped

1 scoop of raw protein powder

1 tsp. of super greens powder

½ a tsp. of ground cinnamon

¼ tsp. of grated ginger

1 tsp. of coconut oil

Water

Directions

1. Place all the ingredients in a blender and top up with water.

2. Blend until smooth.

Minty Maca Smoothie

Ingredients

2 tbsp. hemp of chia seeds

1 tbsp. cacao nibs

1 tbsp. maca powder

1 scoop of raw protein powder

1 scoop of super greens powder

A small handful of mint leaves

2 large handfuls of ice

Water

Directions

1. Place all the ingredients in a blender and top up with water.
2. Blend until smooth.

Detox Smoothie

Ingredients

½ large cucumber, chopped

2 large handfuls of kale

1 large handful of spinach

1 handful of fresh parsley

200ml filtered water

1 small handful of ice

¼ tbsp. of grated ginger

1 tsp. of spirulina

1 tsp. chia seeds

Water

Directions

1.   Place all the ingredients in a blender and top up with water.

2.   Blend until smooth.

Immune-Building Smoothie

Ingredients

¼ tbsp. of grated ginger

1 small cucumber, chopped

2 large handfuls of spinach

1 handful of sprouted seeds

200ml filtered water

Water

Directions

1. Place all the ingredients in a blender and top up with water.

2. Blend until smooth.

Hormone Balancing Maca Smoothie

Ingredients

1 stalk of celery

½ a large cucumber

1 head of lettuce, chopped, with the core removed

1 tbsp. of maca powder

½ tsp. of organic matcha powder

1 scoop of raw protein powder

½ tsp cinnamon

1 tbsp. chia seeds

Small handful of ice

200ml raw coconut milk

Optional – 1 tsp cacao nibs

Water

Directions

1. Place all the ingredients in a blender and top up with water.

2. Blend until smooth.

Sweet Potato and Sesame Bliss Smoothie

Ingredients

1 small raw sweet potato, peeled and chopped

200ml of unsweetened almond or other nut or seed milk

1 scoop of raw protein powder

1 tsp. ashwaghanda

1 tsp. maca powder

1 tsp. cinnamon powder

Water

Directions

1. Place all the ingredients in a blender and top up with water or more nut milk.
2. Blend until smooth.

I personally do not recommend juices on a yeast cleanse as they can be high in vegetable sugars, so for this reason you won't find them in this book. Feel free to consume regularly before the Cleanse, during the pre-tox, or afterward.

Teas that Heal

The following teas are some of my favourite healthy and healing tea blends.

Warm Ginger, Lemon & Salt Tea

Alkalizing, detoxifying, stimulating, anti-fungal, and anti-bacterial.

Wormwood, Walnut Leaf, Clove Tea

Anti-fungal, antibacterial, antiviral, and detoxifying (You can add Catnip to this mix).

Ginger, Lemon and/or Orange, Cinnamon, Turmeric, Garlic and Honey

Coughs and colds, immune support, and antiviral.

Elderflower Tea

Coughs and colds, and detoxifying.

Peppermint Tea

Natural stimulant, digestive aid, and expectorant (lemon-grass is also a great addition to peppermint; it's tasty, and aids good digestion as well).

Orange Blossom Tea

Quietens the mind.

Jasmine Tea

Antidepressant, antiseptic, helps with sleep, expectorant, and calming (I use the jasmine flowers to make tea, but you can get jasmine green tea in most health food stores, which has the added benefits of green tea).

Lemon Balm Tea

Calming and antiviral (especially effective for the herpes virus/cold sores, etc).

Borage, Liquorice and Ginseng Tea

Adrenal/hormonal support

Chamomile, Lavender & Rosehip Tea

Aids better and most restful sleep (you only need a couple of small petals of rosehip in each pot, as a little goes along way, and if you consume too much it can actually do the opposite and cause nightmares).

PLEASE NOTE:–

It's very important before using any herbs that you check for side-effects to any medications you may be taking, any health concerns you have, and if you are pregnant or breast feeding.

Try, where possible, to purchase organic, unbleached, and not chemically-sealed teabags if you are not making your teas up from fresh and/or dried herbs, as there are a lot of toxic chemicals in many brands of teabags.

Chapter 11: Fermenting Options

Sauerkraut

Ingredients

1 medium cabbage

1 tbsp. sea salt

Optional:

1 tbsp. caraway, coriander, or fennel seeds

3 tbsp. grated ginger (I highly recommend this addition)

200-300g grated carrot

Directions

1. Remove outer leaves from the cabbage, and set them aside.

2. Shred cabbage. I like to use the grating option of my food processor for this.

3. Shred carrots and ginger (if you're adding these).

4. In a bowl, mix the shredded items with seeds (if you're adding these) and sea salt, then massage together or pound down with a mallet or the end of a rolling pin for 10 minutes.

5. Once the juices have been released, place into a wide-mouthed jar and continue to pound down until juices come up and cover the cabbage. (If this does not happen, add a little fresh water until it covers the cabbage well.) Leave a space of 2 inches at the top.

6. Place a whole cabbage leaf over the top of the shredded cabbage, making sure no air can get to the cabbage underneath. If you have no cabbage leaf, then use a clean weight of some sort to weigh it down.

7. Leave in a dark place at room temperature for around a month. You can eat it after 3 days, but it's much tastier and contains more probiotics if left longer. Transfer to fridge once you open it, or after a month or two.

If you leave it to sit for more than a couple of weeks, you may want to 'burp' it (open the lid a little) to release the built-up pressure from the jar.

Kimchi

Ingredients

1/2 head white cabbage

2 carrots (parsnips also work well)

7-8 red radishes

1 small celeriac (optional)

1 small yellow onion

2-inch square fresh ginger

4 cloves garlic (optional)

1 tsp. dried chilli flakes

1 tbsp. salt

25-50ml filtered water or sauerkraut juice

Directions

1. Using the shredding/grating function on your food processor, or a hand grater, grate all the vegetables.

2. Place all ingredients, except the water, into a large bowl and massage the salt thoroughly through the vegetables.

3. Using either a kraut pounder or the end of a rolling pin, pound down the vegetables until the juices are released. This should take around 10-15 minutes. You can also squeeze the juice from the veggies, which is sometimes easier on the arms.

4. Put the vegetable mixture into the jar(s).

5. If the brine mixture from the vegetables does not completely cover them, top up with water until it does.

6. Put a couple of cabbage leaves on the top of your vegetable mixture and weigh down with a clean, boiled stone, or a kitchen weight. Make sure everything is just under the water/brine level, so that it does not go mouldy.

7. Put the lid on the jar and place in a cupboard for a minimum of 2 weeks, preferably a month. The longer you leave it the better, but if you leave it longer than 6 weeks, you will need to 'burp' the jar. It will taste stronger, the longer you leave it.

8. Once opened, put in the fridge. Use it as a side to just about any hot or cold dish for a super-charged meal.

Note:

You can use just about any vegetables in this recipe, so it's a great way to use up veggies!

Fermented Pickles

Ingredients

1 large carrot, cut into slices

1 red pepper, cut into slices

Half a small cauliflower, cut into half florets

1 clove garlic, crushed and peeled

1 bay leaf

½ tsp. coriander seeds

¼ tsp. black peppercorns

3 tsp. Himalayan or sea salt

Filtered water to cover

1-2 grape/raspberry leaves (optional, to keep veggies crisp)

Directions

1. Place all the ingredients, apart from the water and salt, in a large mason jar.
2. Make sure there is at least 2 inches of space in the top of the jar.
3. Add the salt and then the water to cover all the vegetables.
4. Weigh down the vegetables with a large stone or a bag of water. Make sure everything is below the level of the water.
5. Place the lid on the jar and 'burp', to release the gas from the jar, once a day for the first few days and then once a week after that.
6. This is ready to eat after 5 days but will keep for many weeks, especially if you add the grape/raspberry leaves.
7. Do not eat the grape/raspberry leaves.

Fermented Peppers

Ingredients

2-3 peppers, cored and cut into strips

1 small handful of parsley

1 small garlic clove, peeled

1 tsp. Himalayan or sea salt

Filtered water, to cover

Directions

1. Add the parsley and garlic to a mason jar.
2. Place the peppers all standing upright in the jar. Make sure there are enough peppers so that they are wedged in and won't move anywhere when the liquid is added.
3. Add the salt and then fill with the water until the peppers are completely covered. Makes sure there is a space of at least 2 inches between the water and the top of the jar.
4. If you see any peppers floating, then wedge more pieces in so they cannot move.
5. Make sure to 'burp', release the gas from the jar, every day for the first week and then once a week after that. Once you start eating the peppers, leave the jar in the fridge.
6. These are fine to eat after 5 days or up to a few weeks old.

Picked Onions

Ingredients

300-400g of small shallots/pickling onions, peeled

A small handful of fresh rosemary, parsley, or cumin seeds

1 tbsp. Himalayan or sea salt

Filtered water, to cover

Directions

1. Place any herbs you wish into a large mason jar.

2. Add the salt and then the onions.

3. Fill the jar with water, so that all the onions are covered.

4. Weigh down the onions with a weight, stone, or bag of water.

5. Make sure everything is submerged and that no onions or herbs are floating about on the top of the water.

6. Place some muslin over the top of the jar, and secure in place with an elastic band.

7. These are ready to eat after 2 weeks, or for months beyond this.

8. Once you start to eat from the jar, put a lid on it and place in the fridge.

Carrot and Garlic Fermented Sticks

Ingredients

5-6 carrots, washed and cut into sticks about 4 inches' long

2-3 garlic cloves, peeled

A small handful of fresh dill (optional)

2 tsp. Himalayan or sea salt

Filtered water to cover

Directions

1. Add the dill (if using), garlic, and salt to a mason jar.

2. Wedge the carrot sticks into the jar so that they are all standing up and cannot move or float around once you add the liquid.

3. Add the water and make sure the sticks are fully covered, but that there is still a 2-inch space between the water and the top of the jar.

4. Place the lid on the jar.

5. 'Burp', release the gas from the jar, every day for a week and then weekly after that.

6. These are ready to eat in 5 days, or up to a month.

7. Once you start eating from the jar, place the jar into the fridge.

Fermented Parsnip & Carrot

Ingredients

1-2 parsnips (depending on size), topped and tailed, peeled and cut into 4 inch sticks

1-2 carrots, cut into 4 inch sticks

2 inches of fresh ginger, peeled and sliced

1 tbsp. chilli flakes

1 tsp. Himalayan or sea salt

Filtered water, to cover

Directions

1. Place ginger, chilli flakes, and salt into a mason jar.
2. Place the parsnip and carrot sticks into the jar so they are all standing up on end. Wedge them in as tightly as you can, so that none of the vegetable sticks can float about once you add the liquid.
3. Add the water to cover the sticks fully, but so there is also a 2-inch space between the water and the top of the jar.
4. Secure the lid in place.
5. 'Burp', release the gas from the jar, every day for the first week, and then weekly thereafter.
6. These sticks are ready to eat after 5 days, or for up to a month.
7. Once you start eating from the jar, place it in the fridge.

Fermented Salsa

Ingredients

2 large tomatoes, diced

1 red or green pepper, diced

1 onion, diced

1-2 fresh chillies, chopped

1-2 cloves of garlic, minced

1 handful of parsley or coriander, chopped

2-3 tsp. of Himalayan or sea salt

Filtered water, to cover, if needed

Directions

1. Mix all the ingredients well in a large bowl.
2. Place ingredients into a mason jar.
3. Push the ingredients down in the jar so there is no space around them, and so that some of the liquid is released to cover the ingredients. If the liquid does not cover all the ingredients, place a little extra water in the jar to cover them fully, but allowing there to be a 2-inch space between the liquid and the top of the jar.
4. Secure the lid onto the jar, but only tight enough to stop anything getting in yet still allowing the gas to get out.
5. Check the gas can still escape the following day and, if not, loosen slightly.
6. This salsa can be eaten the very next day, or for up to a month or two later.
7. Once you start eating from it, put the lid on fully and place in the fridge.

Onion Relish

Ingredients

3 or 4 large onions, peeled and sliced thinly, or grated

1-2 tbsp. peppercorns

2 tsp. Himalayan or sea salt

Filtered water, to cover

Directions

1. Place all the ingredients in a large bowl and mix well.
2. Leave covered for 30 minutes, until some of the liquid from the onions has started to collect in the bowl.
3. Place everything (including the liquid) into a mason jar, and press down so that the liquid comes up above the onions. Add a little filtered water if this does not happen.
4. Place the lid firmly on the jar.
5. 'Burp', release the gas from the jar, every day for the first week and then weekly after that.
6. The relish is ready to eat after a week, or for many months thereafter.

Beet Kvass

Ingredients

2-4 fresh beetroots

40-60ml juice from sauerkraut

1 tbsp. Himalayan or sea salt

Filtered water, to cover

Directions

1. Wash beets and peel, if not organic; leave skin on if organic.
2. Chop beets into small cubes: don't grate.
3. Place beets in mason jar.
4. Add sauerkraut juice and salt. (If you don't want to use sauerkraut juice, double the salt. It may take longer to ferment.)
5. Fill jar with filtered water.
6. Cover with muslin and leave on the counter at room temperature for 2 days to ferment.
7. Transfer to fridge.

Milk Kefir

Ingredients

900ml raw milk (or organic whole milk)

1-2 tbsp. milk kefir grains (these are not the same grains as water kefir ones, but can be purchased in the same places)

Directions

1. Place your kefir grains in the mason jar and add the milk.
2. Stir with a wooden spoon (remember, no metal as this can harm the grains), cover and secure with muslin and elastic band, and leave at room temperature to culture for up to 1-3 days, depending on preferred taste or room temperature.
3. A shorter fermentation time will mean a milder flavour, and a longer one will mean a stronger and sourer flavour.
4. Once your kefir is done culturing, remove the grains (this is usually easier with your hands, as it can be quite thick). Store the kefir milk in the refrigerator and begin another batch with the grains.

Note: For this Cleanse program, I haven't included water kefir or kombucha because, if you are not sure what you are doing with them, they could feed a yeast imbalance rather than the opposite, which is what we want.

Sourdough

Ingredients

480g flour (I prefer spelt flour)

100g sourdough starter

220ml fresh water

1 tsp. salt

Directions

1. Mix well 100g of sourdough starter with 300g of flour and 220ml of water in a bowl and cover for 8-10 hours (at this or any of the later stages, you can add herbs, chillies, sundried tomatoes, or other similar items).

2. Add the remaining 180g of flour and the sugar, and knead well. Cover and allow to rest for another 2-3 hours.

3. Knead again and pop into a lightly oiled bread tin or proof basket, cover, and leave in a warm place for 1-2 hours. (You can lightly score the top of the dough at this stage, if you want to.)

4. Preheat your oven on a medium heat (around 350°F/180°C/gas mark 4) and put a bowl of boiling water on the bottom of your oven.

5. Place dough in its baking tin/baking basket in the upper oven, and bake for 30-35 minutes.

6. Remove from the tin and allow it to cool slightly before cutting into it.

Notes:

1. Your sourdough starter needs to be fed once a week, and should live in your fridge until the day before you want to use it.

2. To feed your sourdough starter, add 50g flour and 50ml fresh water. Mix well and pop back in the fridge until you want to use it.

3. Your starter will separate (with the hooch lying on top). This is fine, and it just needs stirring back in each week when you feed it.

Wild Garlic Pesto

Ingredients

700g-1kg wild garlic leaves

120g pine nuts or chopped almonds

1 tbsp. salt

60ml filtered water

50-100g basil leaves

Salt and pepper

Directions

1. Blend all the ingredients, except the water, in a food processor. (You can change the ratio of ingredients to your personal taste.)

2. Add mixture to jar and top up with the water so it comes just above the level of the mixture.

3. Place a small plate or weight over the top of the mixture, so that it is all submerged.

4. Pop the lid on, and put in a cupboard for anywhere between 10 days and 2 months. Place in the fridge once opened.

Notes:

1. You can ferment the wild garlic by itself (as per the above directions), so that you have a store of probiotic garlic to last you through the winter.

2. You can add olive oil to the jar rather than brine/salted water, and this will make a pesto closer to shop-bought pesto, and one that you can use almost straight away.

3. Don't pull up the wild garlic bulbs – the leaves (and flowers) are the best bit of wild garlic, and if you leave the bulbs, even more wild garlic will be there next year.

UK Measurements	USA Measurements
240ml	1 cup
480ml	1 pint
950ml	1 quart
125g flour	1 cup flour
225g butter	1 cup butter
170g sugar	1 cup sugar
90g oats	1 cup uncooked oats
170g rice	1 cup uncooked rice
100g chopped nuts	1 cup chopped nuts
140g dried fruit	1 cup dried fruit

With Love

I couldn't let you leave without a little bit of love! I want you to know you deserve all the goodness you are doing for yourself, and more. And if you don't feel this way about yourself then please, please, please use this as an invitation to resolve that piece of disharmony inside yourself that makes you feel that way.

We did not come to this planet to live in despair, to hate ourselves, or to walk around in total overwhelm. Trust me when I say I know – I've played that game (for most of my life). It's exhausting and it blooming hurts! We are magical beings, flying through an infinite Universe on a giant rotating ball of rock and water! Now what's not to love about that? You are awesome, you are totally different from those around you, and that's what makes you... you, and makes them... them. Spend your time and energy on enjoying being you, and let go of trying to be whoever you think you should be, then watch your energy, love of life, and love of yourself come flooding back to you.

If you are struggling to make nourishing and nurturing choices for yourself, then willpower will only get you so far, and that so far isn't actually very far at all! If you are struggling, see the struggle as an invitation to heal a little more of what's preventing you from living in health, happiness, and harmony. Every sign or symptom from the body is simply another invitation, and when you view your existing or new ailments in this way it helps you to see the perceived issues differently, and to use them to resolve a little something more in your life.

It is my opinion that the only way to become happy, healthy, and harmonious in all areas of your life is to become connected to all areas of your life again. For this reason, be willing to experience all that is happening to you; don't push it away, medicate it, or pretend it's not there, as it's a message from the body that something is out of balance. Conflict within the body causes dis-ease. Clean up the conflict, use the symptom as a means to tap on something out of balance within the body and mind, and invite more happiness, health, and harmony in.

Use the struggle to help you heal. This, by default, allows you to love yourself and your life a little more!

Embrace you – you totally and utterly rock!!!!

With much love,

Faith xx

Books that Heal

Way of the Peaceful Warrior – Dan Millman

Mutant Message Down Under – Marlo Morgan

The Alchemist – Paulo Coelho

The Pilgrimage – Paulo Coelho (or just about anything else by Paulo)

Awareness – Anthony De Mello

The Way to Love – Anthony De Mello

The Power of Now – Eckhart Tolle

A New Earth – Eckhart Tolle

The Celestine Prophecy – James Redfield

A Simple Act of Gratitude – John Kralik

Energy Healing – Abby Wynne

Healing Breakthroughs – Dr. Larry Dossey

The Biology of Belief – Bruce Lipton

It's the Thought that Counts – David Hamilton

How the Mind Can Heal the Body – David Hamilton

Mind Calm – Sandy Newbigging

Body Calm – Sandy Newbigging

Lucid Dreaming – Charlie Morley

The Journey – Brandon Bays

I Can See Clearly Now – Wayne Dyer

The Top Ten Things Dead People Want to Tell You – Mike Dooley

Dying to Be Me – Anita Moorjani

Akashic Records – Gabrielle Orr

Daily Love: Growing Into Grace – Mastin Kipp

The Art of Extreme Self-Care: Transform Your Life One Month at a Time – Cheryl Richardson

Embrace – Taryn Brumfit

Embody – Connie Sobczak

The Happiness Project – Gretchen Rubin

Hector and the Search for Happiness – Francois Lelord

The Unlikely Pilgrimage of Harold Fry – Rachel Joyce

Walking Home – Sonia Choquette

The Camino: A Pilgrimage Of Courage – Shirley MacLaine

Wild: A Journey from Lost to Found (Paperback) – Cheryl Strayed

How to Heal Toxic Thoughts – Sandra Ingerman

Big Magic – Elizabeth Gilbert

Light is the New Black – Rebecca Campbell

Conscious Writing – Julia McCutchen

The Mandala Book – Lori Bailey Cunningham

The Fire Starter Sessions – Danielle Laporte

Creating Mandalas: For Insight, Healing, and Self-Expression Paperback – Susanne F. Fincher

The Art of Non Conformity – Chris Guillebeau

The Happiness of Pursuit – Chris Guillebeau

Low Impact Man – Colin Beavan

Last Child in the Woods – Richard Louv

Earthing: The Most Important Health Discovery Ever – Clinton Ober, Stephen Sinatra, and Martin Zucker

Toxic Childhood: How The Modern World Is Damaging Our Children And What We Can Do About It – Sue Palmer

Joyful Recovery – Sasha Allenby

Longevity Now – David Wolfe

Cultured Food for Life – Donna Schwenk

Is it Me or My Adrenals? – Marcelle Pick

Adrenal Fatigue – James Wilson

The Tapping Solution for Weight Loss and Body Confidence – Jessica Ortner

Raw Food – Ani Phyo

Easy Raw Vegan Dehydrating – Kristen Suzanne

Lightning Source UK Ltd.
Milton Keynes UK
UKOW05f1823270117
293006UK00008B/83/P